PLATINUM
VIGNETTES™

ULTRA-HIGH-YIELD CLINICAL CASE SCENARIOS
FOR USMLE STEP 2

Surgical Subspecialties

ADAM BROCHERT, MD

Resident
Department of Radiology
Medical College of Georgia
Memorial Health University Medical Center
Savannah, Georgia

Hanley & Belfus, Inc. / Philadelphia

Publisher: HANLEY & BELFUS, INC.
               Medical Publishers
               210 South 13th Street
               Philadelphia, PA 19107
               (215) 546-7293; 800-962-1892
               FAX (215) 790-9330
               Web site: http://www.hanleyandbelfus.com

Note to the reader: Although the information in this book has been carefully reviewed for correctness of dosage and indications, neither the author nor the publisher can accept any legal responsibility for any errors or omissions that may be made. Neither the publisher nor the author makes any warranty, expressed or implied, with respect to the material contained herein. Before prescribing any drug, the reader must review the manufacturer's current product information (package inserts) for accepted indications, absolute dosage recommendations, and other information pertinent to the safe and effective use of the product described. This is especially important when drugs are given in combination or as an adjunct to other forms of therapy.

PLATINUM VIGNETTES™: SURGICAL SUBSPECIALTIES   ISBN 1-56053-538-5

Library of Congress Control Number: 2002106492

Last digit is the print number: 9 8 7 6 5 4 3 2 1

INTRODUCTION

Case scenarios are a great way to review for the USMLE Step 2 exam. A high percentage of current exam questions center on case studies or patient presentations in an office or emergency department setting. Practicing this format and being familiar with the majority of the classic, "guaranteed-to-be-on-the-exam" case scenarios gives the examinee an obvious, clear-cut advantage. *Platinum Vignettes*™ were written to offer you that advantage.

You need to be familiar not only with pathophysiology, but also the work-up and management of several conditions to succeed on the USMLE Step 2 exam. Sifting through the history, physical exam findings, and various tests, you are expected to make and confirm the diagnosis and manage the patient's condition.

Each book in the *Platinum Vignettes*™ presents 50 case scenarios or clinical vignettes. The individual vignettes are followed by the diagnosis, pathophysiology, diagnostic strategies, and management issues pertaining to that specific patient. The reader must turn the page to obtain these latter details, and is encouraged to "guess" before reading about the patient's condition and course. In fact, you are advised not only to guess the diagnosis, but also to postulate on which test to order next, what therapy to give, and what to "watch out" for in the condition presented.

Important words or phrases ("buzzwords") are set in bold type in the explanation of each vignette. These words or phrases indicate the material most commonly asked about on the exam or are important in helping to distinguish one condition from another. This format is designed for review of material that was previously learned during rotations; therefore, further reading is advised if the topic or buzzwords are unfamiliar. Remember, buzzwords are rarely helpful unless you know what they mean!

Every attempt was made to provide the most current, up-to-date information on every topic tackled in this volume and every volume in the series—but medicine is a rapidly changing field. If you hear about a new therapy in a conference or on rounds, it may well be that the standard of care has changed. Remember, though, that what you see on the wards and in the office isn't always applicable to the boards (e.g., everyone with pneumonia should not be given the latest "big-gun" antibiotic; all patients with headaches should not receive a CT scan).

Good luck!

ADAM BROCHERT, MD

NOTE: A standard Table of Contents, with cases listed by diagnosis, would give you too much of a head start on solving each patient scenario. Challenge yourself! When ready, you can turn to the detailed Case Index at the back of this book.

Case 1

Ophthalmology

History

A 58-year-old black man presents with a long history of gradually worsening vision in both eyes, the right slightly more affected than the left. The patient has never worn glasses and has never had an eye exam before. He says he is otherwise in good health and has had no other problems with his eyes or vision. His father and grandfather became blind in their 60s, but causes were unknown, as both disliked doctors and never sought a diagnosis. The patient does not take any medications and denies headaches and the use of alcohol or other drugs.

Exam

T: 98.2°F   BP: 144/88   RR: 12/min.   P: 82/min.

The man is slightly overweight, but otherwise appears healthy and is in no acute distress. Visual acuity is 20/25 bilaterally, with decreased peripheral vision bilaterally on visual field examination. Pupillary and corneal exams are unremarkable. No conjunctival injection is appreciated. Funduscopic exam reveals abnormal-looking optic discs, with increased cup-to-disc ratios and a "scooped out" appearance of the central cups. The blood vessels passing over the margin of the optic nerve head are nasally displaced (see figure). The remainder of the funduscopic exam is unremarkable. Tonometry reveals ocular pressure of 38 mmHg in the right eye and 34 mmHg in the left eye (normal < 22 mmHg).

Tests

Hemoglobin: 15 g/dL (normal 14–18)
White blood cell (WBC) count: 7200/μL (normal 4500–11,000)
Creatinine: 1.1 mg/dL (normal 0.6–1.5)

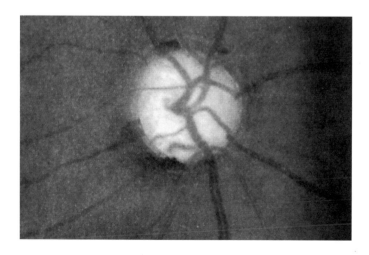

Glaucoma, open-angle type

The figure shows enlargement of the optic cup ("optic cupping") with an increased cup-to-disc ratio.

Pathophysiology

Glaucoma is best thought of as **ocular hypertension** with resultant visual loss. Its pathophysiology is complex and heterogeneous. Two primary clinical types are **open-angle** and **closed-angle** (or narrow-angle). Open-angle glaucoma (OAG) causes **90%** of cases and is often **asymptomatic for years** until vision loss occurs, while closed-angle (CAG) accounts for **10%** of cases and usually presents in a dramatic, acute fashion. Glaucoma can be primary or secondary to **trauma, cataracts, or inflammation.** The primary risk factors are **age > 40, black race, family history, chronic steroid use, severe myopia, and diabetes.** Roughly 2% of adults over age 40 are affected in the U.S., and **screening at least every 3 years** after this age is advised, with more aggressive screening for higher-risk persons.

Diagnosis & Treatment

Physicians must screen for OAG with **tonometry** (a way to measure intraocular pressure), because it is usually asymptomatic initially. Some patients may complain of **occasional, transient blurring of vision.** CAG presents with **sudden ocular pain (one or both eyes), decreased vision, a red eye, seeing halos around lights, and nausea and vomiting.**

On exam, OAG patients generally have **increased intraocular pressure** (> 20–22 mmHg). In more advanced disease, there may be **"cupping" of the optic disc,** which may be **pale,** with an **increased cup-to-disc ratio** and nasal displacement of the optic vessels. **Visual acuity is often normal** until fairly late in the disease, with **visual field deficits** (first in the nasal fields, then the temporal fields) occuring first. CAG patients presenting during an "attack" (which doesn't occur in open-angle patients) have a **red eye with corneal clouding, decreased visual acuity, markedly increased intraocular pressure (> 30–40 mmHg) and a fixed, mid-dilated pupil.**

In OAG patients, treatment is generally eye drops (e.g., **beta blockers, prostaglandins,** acetazolamide, or pilocarpine). Patients are followed with periodic computerized **visual field testing.** If drugs fail (progressive visual field loss) or if patients dislike or are noncompliant with medications, surgery is an option. *In CAG patients,* **surgery is a first-line treatment** (peripheral laser iridectomy). However, an acute attack in a CAG patient is an emergency that may result in blindness *within hours* if not treated, and drugs such as pilocarpine, acetazolamide, and oral glycerin are used to "break" the attack prior to surgery.

More High-Yield Facts

Anticholinergics can trigger glaucoma attacks *only in CAG patients who have never received treatment,* not in OAG or CAG patients previously treated with surgery.

Case 2

Ophthalmology

History

A 42-year-old man is troubled by sudden, painless visual loss in his right eye. He says it felt like "a curtain came down" over his eye a few hours ago. He also describes seeing flashes of light in addition to several tiny black spots in front of his eye; they seem to stay in his field of view no matter where he looks. The patient denies problems in his left eye. He is nearsighted and wears glasses, but has had a stable prescription for 10 years and no visual complaints before today. He has no significant past medical history and takes no medications or other drugs. There is no family history of visual problems other than nearsightedness.

Exam

T: 98.5°F   BP: 124/78   RR: 14/min.   P: 72/min.

The patient is in no acute distress and appears healthy. While he is wearing his glasses, visual acuity is 20/20 bilaterally, with decreased vision in the superior field of the right eye on visual field examination. Pupillary, conjunctival, and corneal exams are unremarkable. Funduscopic exam reveals normal optic discs bilaterally. Tonometry demonstrates normal ocular pressure bilaterally.

Tests

Erythrocyte sedimentation rate (ESR): 8 mm/hr (normal 1–20)
MRI of the brain: negative

Pathophysiology

Retinal detachment may be idiopathic or can occur after **trauma/eye surgery,** from **proliferative retinopathy** (e.g., diabetes or sickle cell disease), or from ocular tumors or severe inflammation (e.g., uveitis). It is commonly **associated with myopia** as well. The degree of visual impairment depends on the location and extent of the retinal tear.

Diagnosis & Treatment

The classic patient history is **painless, sudden loss of vision,** typically described as a **curtain or veil coming into the field of vision.** Initially seeing **flashing lights** followed by "**floaters,**" or small dark spots in the field of vision no matter where one looks, is also classic.

Visual acuity may be normal or reduced, depending on whether or not the macula is affected by the tear. Peripheral vision is often affected. The tear *may or may not be visible* on routine indirect ophthalmoscopy. If seen, **retinal irregularity and/or elevation with darkened blood vessels** is typical. Hemorrhage into the vitreous, common in trauma/post-surgical states or with proliferative retinopathy, may totally obscure visualization.

Suspected retinal detachment is an **ophthalmologic emergency** and your job (assuming you're not the ophthalmologist) is to *refer the patient to an ophthalmologist immediately.* The treatment is **surgical,** through various means (e.g., reattachment with photocoagulation or cryopexy, scleral buckling), and reattachment of the retina often is possible. This may allow restoration of vision or, at least, stop the tear from extending and causing further vision loss.

More High-Yield Facts

Other common causes of unilateral, painless loss of vision:
• **Central retinal artery occlusion**—cherry-red spot on the fovea, often associated with temporal arteritis; no good treatment (give steroids with temporal arteritis to prevent blindness in other eye)
• **Transient ischemic attack** (or a stroke)—carotid bruit on affected side is classic; vision usually comes back within an hour if due to a TIA
• **Optic neuritis/papillitis**—often takes several hours to occur and usually causes pain, but sometimes happens quickly and is painless. Look for **blurred disc margins,** which can be a sign of papillitis (inflamed optic disc) or increased intracranial pressure.
• **Conversion reaction**—classic is young female with a normal eye exam who just got in a fight with a family member or boyfriend.

Ophthalmology

History

A 62-year-old man is in your office for a routine follow-up exam. You are following him for type II diabetes, which he was diagnosed with approximately 10 years ago. He is fairly noncompliant. The patient has no current complaints and says he has been taking his medication as prescribed. He is currently on metformin, pioglitazone, and acarbose. Past medical history is otherwise unremarkable.

Exam

T: 98.5°F   BP: 124/76   RR: 14/min.   P: 78/min.

Visual acuity is 20/25 on the right and 20/30 on the left. Visual field examination reveals no deficits. Pupillary, conjunctival, and corneal exams are unremarkable. Funduscopic exam reveals specific changes in both retinas (see figure). Tonometry demonstrates normal ocular pressure bilaterally.

Tests

Hemoglobin A1c: 9.1% (normal < 6%)
ESR: 10 mm/hr (normal 1–20)
Urinalysis: trace proteinuria; otherwise negative

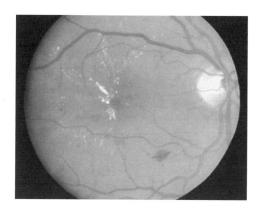

Diabetic retinopathy, background or nonproliferative type

The figure reveals **exudates, dot and blot hemorrhages,** and **edema,** classic changes of diabetic retinopathy.

Pathophysiology

Diabetes is a *leading cause of blindness* (especially in those **under age 50**). The duration of diabetes and degree of long-term diabetic control is correlated with the development of retinopathy. Diabetes-induced microvascular disease with resultant **loss of capillary integrity** is responsible for many of the early retinal changes. Eventually, localized ischemia from microvascular disease results in the release of growth factors, which cause new blood vessels to form (**neovascularity**), many of which are abnormal and prone to bleed. At this point, the retinopathy is said to be *proliferative*. There is a strong association (not a causal link, however) between **proteinuria** and diabetic retinopathy.

Diagnosis & Treatment

Diabetic patients should be **screened annually with a formal ophthalmologic exam—starting at the time of diagnosis for those with type II diabetes, and 5 years after diagnosis for type I diabetes.** Early stages of retinopathy are asymptomatic. As the disease progresses, macular edema may occur, resulting in visual loss that can be fairly sudden.

On exam, the fundus may have **exudates** (which are classically "hard," but may be "soft," cotton-wool spots), **dot and/or blot hemorrhages, microaneurysms,** and **arteriovenous "nicking." Edema** is also common, and may be the cause of recent vision loss if in the macula. Neovascularity, which often occurs near the disc but can be in the peripheral retina, is the hallmark of proliferative retinopathy and indicates advanced disease.

The best treatment for nonproliferative/background retinopathy is **tight control of blood glucose,** which has been shown to delay the development and progression of retinopathy. If macular edema develops, **focal laser** is a preferred treatment. If neovascularity occurs, a procedure known as **panretinal photocoagulation** is used. This involves making several small burns in the periphery of the entire retina with a laser, which is thought to destroy the hypoxic tissue that sent out the signals responsible for inducing neovascularity.

More High-Yield Facts

Hypertension can cause retinopathy that resembles diabetic retinopathy with "cotton-wool" spots ("soft" exudates), arteriovenous nicking, and focal hemorrhages, but **arteriolar narrowing** and **"copper" or "silver" wiring of vessels** are more unique to hypertension.

Ophthalmology

History

A 41-year-old woman is experiencing double vision that came on over the last few days and seems to be getting worse. The patient says her double vision is worst when she tries to look to her left. She denies any previous history of vision problems. She is otherwise in good health and has no significant past medical history, though she does mention fairly frequent headaches that began a few weeks ago. She denies fever or photophobia. Family history is noncontributory and the woman does not smoke, drink alcohol, or use other drugs. She has no history of trauma or psychiatric problems.

Exam

T: 98.5°F   BP: 116/74   RR: 14/min.   P: 68/min.

The woman appears healthy and is alert and oriented. You notice slight lateral and inferior deviation of her right eye at rest, compared to the right. Mild ptosis of the right eyelid is also apparent. In addition, the right pupil is dilated compared to the left and does not constrict normally to light or accomodation. When you ask the patient to turn her right eye inward toward her nose, she cannot adduct it beyond the midline. Funduscopic examination is unremarkable, with sharp optic disks bilaterally. The remainder of the exam is unremarkable, and no other focal neurologic deficits are appreciated.

Tests

Hemoglobin: 15 g/dL (normal 12–16)
WBCs: 6900/μL (normal 4500–11,000)
Platelets: 225,000/μL (normal 150,000–400,000)
ESR: 6 mm/hr (normal 1–15)

Cranial nerve III (oculomotor) palsy with pupillary involvement

Pathophysiology

Third cranial nerve (CN) palsies can be caused by a myriad of disease processes, including **stroke, infection, trauma, microvascular disease** (e.g., from hypertension or diabetes), **tumors, aneurysms,** and **autoimmune** or demyelinating processes. The oculomotor nerve innervates all extraocular muscles except the superior oblique (4th CN) and lateral rectus (6th CN) muscles; innervates the levator palpebrae muscle (thus lesions can cause mild ptosis); and supplies parasympathetic fibers that cause pupillary constriction.

Diagnosis & Treatment

Patients with 3rd CN paralysis complain of **double vision** (i.e., diplopia) that gets *worse* when they try to adduct the affected eye toward the nose. Associated symptoms may be present due to the underlying cause (e.g., headache with a tumor or anuerysm).

On exam, **the eye looks slightly "down and out"** due to the unopposed actions of the lateral rectus and superior oblique. **Mild ptosis** is generally present (the sympathetic chain innervates the tarsal muscles, preventing severe ptosis), and the patient *cannot adduct the affected eye beyond the midline* (due to **medial rectus paralysis**).

With an isolated oculomotor lesion, you must distinguish between "probably benign" 3rd CN lesions and potentially serious causes. If the **pupil is spared** (i.e., normal), the cause is often ischemic, usually secondary to microvascular disease from hypertension and/or diabetes. The pupillary fibers travel superficially in the oculomotor nerve and are more likely to be affected by a space-occupying lesion compressing the nerve, often a **posterior communicating artery aneurysm** or **tumor.** Thus, **a 3rd nerve palsy with a "blown" pupil** (i.e., dilated and nonreactive) **is considered an emergency.**

For isolated 3rd nerve lesions with pupillary sparing and no other symptoms, treatment depends on the patient's situation. If the patient has hypertension and/or diabetes and is over age 40, **observation** is often the mainstay of treatment, with **resolution expected in 4–8 weeks.** With pupillary involvement, a young patient, or no history of hypertension or diabetes, an **MRI/MRA of the brain and intracranial vessels is needed** to rule out aneurysm or tumor.

More High-Yield Facts

Strokes and tumors usually involve more than one cranial nerve.

A blown pupil in the setting of trauma suggests **uncal herniation** from massively increased intracranial pressure.

Ophthalmology

History

A 37-year-old woman complains of a reddened, painful left eye. She also says her eye is sensitive to light and it feels "scratchy," as though there is something in the eye. The patient says these symptoms appeared yesterday, when she began experiencing fever and malaise, and her eye symptoms have been getting progressively worse. She denies any history of similar symptoms as well as fever, skin lesions, right eye symptoms, or sick contacts. The patient has no history of visual problems or other medical problems and takes no medications.

Exam

T: 98.8°F   BP: 118/70   RR: 14/min.   P: 70/min.

The woman is clearly uncomfortable and prefers to keep her left eye shut, saying that the light irritates her eye. You note lacrimation and conjuctival hyperemia of the left eye, as well as a few scattered vesicles on the left eyelid. No foreign body can be identified. Preauricular adenopathy is evident, primarily on the left. Funduscopic examination is normal. The right eye is unremarkable. The appearance of the left eye after topical application of fluorescein is abnormal (see figure). The remainder of the physical examination is unremarkable.

Tests

Hemoglobin: 14 g/dL (normal 12–16)
WBCs: 7300/µL (normal 4500–11,000)
Platelets: 255,000/µL (normal 150,000–400,000)

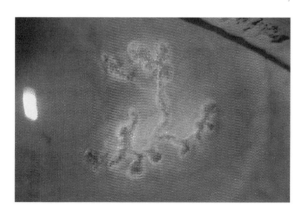

Herpes simplex keratitis

The figure shows classic branching dendritic epithelial ulcers, with terminal bulbs, on the cornea.

Pathophysiology

Herpes simplex keratitis is a corneal infection (from the **type I virus,** not a sexually transmitted disease) and can be primary or due to reactivation of a latent infection. Multiple **recurrences are common,** as with cold sores, and may be brought about by **stress, sunlight, fever,** or **immunosuppression.**

Diagnosis & Treatment

Primary infections tend to cause more systemic symptoms—including **fever, malaise,** and **preauricular adenopathy**—than do recurrences. Eye symptoms include **photophobia, red eye, eye pain,** and **excessive lacrimation.** Initially, patients may have a **vesicular lid eruption,** and vesicular skin lesions occasionally occur around the eye or mouth.

On exam, the hallmark sign is the **branching corneal dendrite,** a collection of classically **confluent branching epithelial ulcers with terminal bulbs.** The **edges of the ulcer usually stain intensely with fluorescein.** Fluorescein is a fluorescent dye used to examine the cornea for ulcerations/epithelial defects, which take up the stain and allow easier visualization.

A herpes eye infection should prompt **ophthalmologic referral.** Treatment is with **antiviral eye drops** (e.g., trifluorothymidine). **Don't give topical steroids if corneal dendrites are present** as you may make things worse.

More High-Yield Facts

Herpes zoster can also cause keratitis similar to herpes simplex keratitis, but skin lesions will be in a classic dermatomal distribution (V_1 **segment of trigeminal nerve** on one side of the face, without crossing the midline), often involving the **tip of the nose** (called Hutchinson's sign, indicates probable ocular involvement). Herpes zoster corneal dendrites do *not* have terminal bulbs and do *not* stain well with fluorescein. Treatment is with **oral acyclovir** (or an analog, e.g., valacyclovir).

Bacterial, fungal, and amebic corneal ulcers can also occur and often present with a roundish, whitish or yellowish (purulent-appearing) lesion on the cornea. *Immediate ophthalmologic referral* is needed to prevent blindness. Corneal scraping for culture is obtained before starting empiric antibiotics. In contact lens wearers, *Pseudomonas* or *Acanthamoeba* are classic causes.

Exposure to **ultraviolet light** (e.g., tanning bed/sunlamp, welders, snow-skiing) can cause keratitis with same symptoms as other forms of keratitis. History helps; no ulcers are seen with fluorescein. Treat with **eye patch** (24 hours) and **topical antibiotic.** Symptoms should resolve **within 48 hours.**

Ophthalmology

History

A 49-year-old man comes into the office complaining of gradual vision loss in both eyes. The patient says his symptoms began several months ago and his vision has been slowly getting worse, to the point where he can no longer tolerate it. He denies pain, fever, or other symptoms and is usually in good health. He says his near vision is primarily affected. Past medical history is significant for hypertension and osteoarthritis of the right knee from a colleakage football injury. The patient takes enalapril, metoprolol, and celecoxib. There is no family history of blindness.

Exam

T: 98.1°F   BP: 148/92   RR: 14/min.   P: 80/min.

The patient is slightly overweight. Visual acuity is 20/20 in the right eye and 20/25 in the left eye. You hand him a magazine to read and he has trouble making out the words. You notice that he tries to hold the magazine as far as away from his eyes as he can in an attempt to make out the letters. The pupils are equally round and reactive to light and accomodation. A normal red reflex is noted. No corneal or conjunctival abnormalities are appreciated. Funduscopic exam reveals mild arteriovenous nicking and a "copper wire" appearance to the fundal arteries. Intraocular pressure is normal bilaterally.

Tests

Hemoglobin: 16 g/dL (normal 14–18)
WBCs: 8300/μL (normal 4500–11,000)
Platelets: 305,000/μL (normal 150,000–400,000)
ESR: 7 mm/hr (normal 0–20)

Incidental mild hypertensive retinopathy is also present.

Pathophysiology

Presbyopia refers to a **loss of the ability to accommodate** that occurs with aging, because the lens gradually becomes less pliable and cannot increase in thickness in response to the action of the ciliary muscles. Thus, near vision is affected, but distance vision remains normal. Presbyopia usually occurs between the **ages of 40 and 50** and is almost universal by the age of 50. It is a normal part of aging, *not* a disease.

Diagnosis & Treatment

A **gradual, painless worsening of near vision only** is often manifested by an *inability to read material held in one's hand*. Initially, people may learn to adapt by holding materials at arm's length (i.e., further away from their eyes, reducing the need for accommodation), but usually this compensation becomes inadequate. Distance vision is *unaffected*.

Diagnosis is straightforward in the right age group when only near vision is affected. Treatment is with **corrective ("reading") glasses** (i.e., a **convex** or "plus" lens, often in the form of bifocals), which can be purchased over the counter at most drug stores. Refractive eye surgery (e.g., LASIK) *cannot* currently correct presbyopia.

Always check intraocular pressure to exclude **glaucoma,** and examine the pupillary red reflex to exclude **cataracts,** in any adult patient with a complaint of gradual bilateral loss of vision. **Macular degeneration** and **diabetic retinopathy** are other common etiologies of gradually progressive, painless vision loss.

More High-Yield Facts

Anticholinergic medications can cause paralysis of accommodation (**cycloplegia**), resulting in presbyopia-like symptoms. The classic offenders are **antipsychotics,** but other drugs with anticholinergic properties (e.g., tricyclic antidepressants) can also cause cycloplegia. This property of anticholinergic medications (e.g., tropicamide, homatropine, or atropine eye drops) is exploited by ophthalmologists to dilate and "fix" the pupils, permitting easier and more complete funduscopic visualization. These drops can also help *relieve pain* when the eye is inflamed (e.g., uveitis, keratitis).

Subconjunctival hemorrhages may occur **spontaneously** or after minor trauma. Exam reveals **gross hemorrhage beneath the conjunctiva.** Though the appearance may worry patients (and board examinees), these lesions are usually of *no significance* and *go away in a few weeks*. Treatment is **reassurance.**

Ophthalmology

History

A 68-year-old woman is brought to the office by her husband due to gradual vision loss in both eyes. She says her symptoms began several months ago and her vision continues to get worse. The patient denies pain, fever, or other symptoms and is otherwise in good health. Past medical history is significant for osteoporosis. The patient takes raloxifene and does not smoke or drink alcohol. Family history is remarkable for glaucoma in the patient's uncle.

Exam

T: 98.4°F   BP: 128/80   RR: 16/min.   P: 82/min.

The patient is thin and pleasant. Visual acuity is 20/200 in the right eye and 20/400 in the left eye, and cannot be significantly corrected with refraction. The pupils are equally round and reactive to light and accommodation. The pupillary red reflex is normal. No gross visual field defects are appreciated, and the extraocular muscles are intact. No corneal or conjunctival abnormalities are evident. Intraocular pressure is normal. Funduscopic exam reveals similar appearance of both eyes (see figure). The remainder of the exam is unremarkable.

Tests

ESR: 9 mm/hr (normal 0–15)
Glucose: 78 mg/dL (normal fasting 70–110)

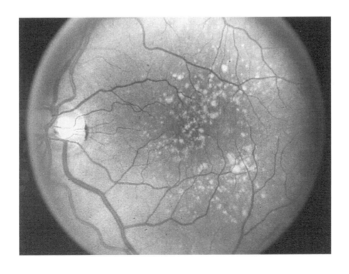

Macular degeneration, age-related

The figure reveals numerous, yellowish-white focal deposits, called **drusen,** in the retina.

Pathophysiology

In the U.S., age-related macular degeneration (ARMD) is one of **the leading causes of significant irreversible visual loss in those over age 50.** The cause is deposition of metabolic by-products, known as drusen, in the retina. Most of these deposits are centered in the macula, the area of highest visual acuity, located lateral to the optic disc. The macula can be identified because it **lacks retinal vessels** (the macula is in the center of the arcade of retinal blood vessels to the right of the disc, centrally located in the figure).

Two main categories of ARMD are recognized clinically: the **"dry" or nonexudative** form and the **"wet" or exudative** form. In the exudative form, hemorrhage and exudation into the retina occur via "leaky" capillaries that result from **neovascularization;** this doesn't occur in the nonexudative form. *The primary risk factor for ARMD is age,* with the incidence increasing sharply after the age of 55.

Diagnosis & Treatment

A **gradual, painless loss of vision** is typical and usually affects both eyes, though often asymmetrically. Because the macula is damaged, visual acuity is primarily affected, and **peripheral vision is often spared,** allowing those affected to perform many activities of daily living even though legally blind in many cases.

Diagnosis is usually made based primarily on the funduscopic appearance and clinical history. The ophthalmologist characterizes the type of ARMD with the aid of a test known as **fluorescein angiography,** which involves injecting fluorescein dye intravenously and taking photos of the retinal vessels. If the exudative type is present (much less common), therapy with **laser photocoagulation** or **photodynamic therapy** with **verteporfin** may be of benefit. For those with the more common nonexudative ARMD, treatment is primarily supportive, employing "low-vision" devices (e.g., magnification aids, special spectacles).

More High-Yield Facts

Corrective lenses *cannot* restore visual acuity because the macula has been damaged. With cataracts, lenses can often correct vision to some extent.

Medications and toxins can also cause vision loss. The classic example is **methanol poisoning,** but **thioridazine, ethambutol, and hydroxychloroquine** can all cause vision loss.

Ophthalmology

History

A 66-year-old woman is troubled by fatigue, muscular weakness, and a unilateral headache on the right side. She also mentions that she is having trouble seeing out of her right eye this morning. The patient has experienced nagging pain, stiffness, and weakness in her neck, shoulder, and hip muscles, accompanied by generalized fatigue and "just feeling lousy," for the last few months. The headaches began a week ago and are only only the right side; her right forehead is tender when she brushes her hair. The patient states that markedly decreased vision in her right eye, which began just a few hours ago, was what finally brought her in to see you. Her past medical history is unremarkable, and the only medication she takes is acetaminophen to relieve her current musculoskeletal symptoms. Family history is non-contributory. The patient does not smoke or drink alcohol, and denies feeling sad or suicidal.

Exam

T: 100.2°F   BP: 132/84   RR: 16/min.   P: 86/min.

The patient is thin, but appears well nourished. Visual acuity is 20/25 in the left eye, but she can barely discern motion with the right eye. The funduscopic appearance of the right eye is abnormal (see figure); the left eye is normal. No photophobia is present, and the intraocular pressures are normal. The patient's right scalp is tender to palpation. Muscle strength is normal in all muscle groups. The remainder of the examination is unremarkable.

Tests

Hemoglobin: 10 g/dL (normal 12–16)
Ferritin: 320 μg/L (normal 20–200)
WBCs: 11,300/μL (normal 4500–11,000)
Platelets: 415,000/μL (normal 150,000–400,000)
ESR: 119 mm/hr (normal 0–15)

Mean corpuscular volume (MCV):
    88 μm/cell (normal 80–100)

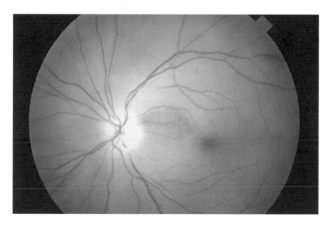

Temporal arteritis and central retinal artery occlusion, with associated polymyalgia rheumatica

The figure reveals the classic **"cherry-red spot" in the macula,** indicating central retinal artery occlusion (though a cherry-red spot can also be seen in **Tay-Sach's disease**).

Pathophysiology

Temporal arteritis (TA)—cranial arteritis or giant-cell arteritis—is a vasculitis that typically affects those **over age 50,** with a *slight female preponderance.* The arteries of the carotid system, especially the cranial arteries, are classically involved, but the aorta and its other branches can also be affected by the characteristic **granulomatous inflammation** that usually includes **giant cells** histologically. **Polymyalgia rheumatica** (PR) commonly occurs in those with TA, though *most patients with PR never develop TA.* PR is a poorly understood myalgic syndrome. Central retinal artery occlusion is a rare but dreaded complication of TA (though it can be due to other etiologies or idiopathic) that often results in blindness.

Diagnosis & Treatment

The classic history for someone with TA is a **unilateral headache,** often **severe,** described as **throbbing** and in the **scalp or temporal region. Scalp tenderness** is also classic (e.g., hurts when patient brushes his or her hair). Jaw pain when eating or talking (**jaw claudication**) is also classic. Visual disturbances are feared (though fairly uncommon) and include **amaurosis fugax, blurry vision, and diplopia.** Systemic symptoms are related to PR and include **fatigue; malaise;** and **pain, stiffness** (especially in the morning), and **weakness** affecting the muscles of the **neck** and **pectoral** and **pelvic regions.** Weight loss and depression may occur.

On exam, scalp tenderness with **swelling and nodularity** in the region of the temporal artery are classic. Muscle strength is usually *normal.* The classic laboratory abnormality is a **markedly elevated ESR** (often > 100 mm/hr), which can be seen with isolated TA or PR. A normocytic **anemia of chronic disease** is also common in both conditions.

In the setting of suspected TA, **corticosteroids should be started immediately—before the diagnosis is confirmed—to prevent blindness** (or in this case, to prevent bilateral blindness). The diagnosis can be confirmed later with a **temporal artery biopsy.** Isolated PR is often clinically diagnosed in the appropriate setting after serology for other autoimmune disorders is negative and electromyography and/or muscle biopsy is normal. Treatment for PR is also with corticosteroids.

More High-Yield Facts

There is *no* satisfactory treatment for central retinal artery occlusion.

Ophthalmology

History

A 72-year-old man seeks medical advice for gradual loss of vision in both eyes that began several months ago. The patient wears reading glasses, but otherwise had no problems with his eyes prior to the current complaint. He denies pain, but says he feels as though he is "looking through a dirty windshield." Past medical history is remarkable for hypertension and gout. The patient takes atenolol and as-needed colchicine for gouty attacks. Family history is noncontributory.

Exam

T: 98.6°F   BP: 130/84   RR: 14/min.   P: 68/min.

Visual acuity is 20/40 in the right eye and 20/60 in the left. With refraction, 20/20 vision can be achieved in both eyes. The pupils are equally round and reactive to light and accommodation. No corneal or conjunctival abnormalities are appreciated. Dark defects are noted in the pupillary red reflex bilaterally. The extraocular muscles are intact, and no visual field deficits are evident. Intraocular pressure is normal bilaterally. Funduscopic exam is limited, because of poor visualization of the fundus. The remainder of the exam is unremarkable, with no focal neurologic deficits or adenopathy noted.

Tests

Hemoglobin: 16 g/dL (normal 14–18)
WBCs: 7100/μL (normal 4500–11,000)
Platelets: 280,000/μL (normal 150,000–400,000)
ESR: 10 mm/hr (normal 0–20)

Pathophysiology

Cataracts are opacities of the lens of the eye, which can be **developmental** or **degenerative.** Most are degenerative and related to **aging.** Other conditions that increase the risk of cataracts in adults include **diabetes, corticosteroid use,** and **inflammation** (e.g., **uveitis**).

Diagnosis & Treatment

Cataracts are one of the common causes of **gradually progressive, painless loss of vision.** Though often **bilateral,** cataracts commonly affect one eye more than the other. Patients typically describe a feeling of "**looking through a dirty windshield.**" Bright lights may cause glare, and *difficulty driving at night* (due to bright oncoming headlights) is fairly common. With a complaint of difficulty driving at night, don't forget to consider possible **vitamin A deficiency.**

On exam, the classic finding is a **dark defect in the pupillary red reflex,** though many cataracts are identified by the naked eye because a **grey or white opacity** is evident on the lens. Patients with cataracts often develop **myopia** due to enlargement of the lens from the cataract and in some cases will **no longer need reading glasses** secondary to the increased refractive power of the enlarged lens. This can lead patients to the classic, false conclusion that their eyes are "getting stronger." Typically, those with cataracts can achieve **improved vision with refractive lenses,** unlike those with glaucoma or retinal diseases.

Management is conservative initially, with **corrective glasses or lenses.** The patient's prescription may *change fairly often* as the cataract continues to enlarge. Once the degree of reduced visual function interferes with the patient's activities of daily living, **surgical removal of the lens** and implantation of a prosthetic lens is the treatment of choice.

More High-Yield Facts

Congenital cataracts are uncommon, but classically occur due to **intrauterine infections** (classically **rubella,** but also toxoplasmosis and cytomegalovirus); **galactosemia;** or **chromosomal abnormalities** (e.g., **Down or Turner syndrome**). They can also be *inherited* (autosomal dominant) or *idiopathic.* Treatment is often surgical to prevent **amblyopia.**

In older children and adolescents, cataracts usually are due to secondary causes, such as **corticosteroid use** (e.g., juvenile rheumatoid arthritis patients) or **diabetes.**

Ophthalmology

History

A 3-year-old child is brought in for a routine visit by his mother. The mother states that the child has no problems; has been "happy and healthy"; and has been growing and developing quickly. The child eats a wide variety of foods and has no significant past medical history. He takes no medications, and his vaccinations are up-to-date. Family history is unremarkable.

Exam

T: 98.7°F   BP: 90/60   RR: 14/min.   P: 94/min.

The child is well developed and appears healthy. Height and weight are appropriate for age. The pupils are equally round and reactive to light and accommodation. No corneal or conjunctival abnormalities are appreciated. When you examine his pupillary light reflex on the left, you notice an unusual appearance (see figure, *left*). The right pupillary light reflex is normal. The extraocular muscles are intact. Visual acuity is decreased on the left compared to the right. The remainder of the examination is normal.

Tests

Hemoglobin: 12 g/dL (normal 11–13)
WBCs: 7900/μL (normal 6000–16,000)

CT scan of a different patient with the same condition in the right eye: see figure, *right*.

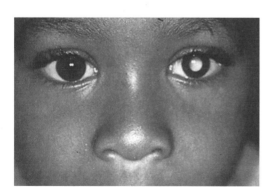

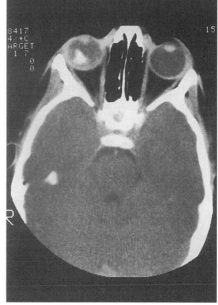

Retinoblastoma

The photo demonstrates leukocoria in the left eye. The CT scan shows a calcified (white) mass in the posterior aspect of the right globe (on the left side of the image).

Pathophysiology

Retinoblastoma is a rare malignant tumor of the retina that usually affects children **between 1 and 2 years of age.** It is the **most common eye malignancy in children.** The pathophysiology is interesting, as identifiable genetic mutations, which can be spontaneous or inherited, are thought to be responsible for the development of the malignancy.

Diagnosis & Treatment

The classic presentation is **leukocoria,** or a change in the normal pupillary **red reflex to white.** Children may also have **strabismus** (a "lazy eye"). When leukocoria or strabismus is noted on exam, *referral to an ophthalmologist is indicated.* The most common cause of leukocoria is **cataracts,** but retinoblastoma is the feared (and classic) etiology for this finding, especially when **unilateral and associated with strabismus.**

When the tumor is **bilateral** (roughly **30% of cases**), the age of presentation is **less than 1 year**, or there is a **family history** of retinoblastoma, the child has most likely *inherited* the **autosomal dominant mutation** responsible for the tumor. Genetic counseling is important in this setting, as both the child and his or her parents have a high risk of affected offspring. Older children with unilateral disease often have a *spontaneous* mutation.

Pathologic diagnosis and treatment are beyond the scope of the Step 2 exam. The CT scan shows the classic appearance. **Survival is high (90–95%),** with vision preservation the most pressing concern in cases of bilateral involvement. Surgical removal of the eye is often employed for unilateral tumors. Children are at risk for **secondary malignancies** later in life, classically **osteosarcoma** in adolescence, due to the cancer susceptibility caused by the same genetic mutation responsible for the retinoblastoma (on **chromosome 13**).

More High-Yield Facts

Leukocoria or persistent strabismus should prompt *referral to an ophthalmologist.*

The most common eye malignancy in adults is **metastatic.** The most common primary malignancy is **malignant melanoma.**

Ophthalmology

History

A 6-year-old child is brought to the emergency department for fever as well as pain and redness in and around his left eye. He had been doing well until 5 days ago, when he developed a greenish-yellow nasal discharge and low-grade fever. The patient's mother treated the child with acetaminophen and over-the-counter sinus medications. Yesterday, some swelling and redness of the left eyelid developed. This morning, he began to complain of pain in his left eye and blurry vision.

The child has a history of sinusitis in the past, but medical history is otherwise unremarkable. He has never had vision problems in the past and does not wear glasses. Family history is noncontributory, and the mother says her son is otherwise healthy and well adjusted. Vaccinations are up-to-date.

Exam

T: 102°F   BP: 96/62   RR: 18/min.   P: 112/min.

The child's left eyelid is swollen and erythematous, with obvious conjunctival injection and edema in the left eye. The left eye is also mildly proptotic compared to the right. The pupils are equally round and reactive to light and accommodation. Extraocular muscles are intact on the right, but he has a globally decreased range of motion in the left eye, in part due to pain. Visual acuity is 20/20 in the right eye and 20/80 in the left eye. No adenopathy is appreciated in the head and neck. You note a greenish-yellow nasal discharge and mild tachycardia, but the remainder of the exam is unremarkable.

Tests

Hemoglobin: 12 g/dL (normal 11–13)
WBCs: 16,500/μL (normal 5000–14,500)
Neutrophils: 86%
Platelets: 390,000/μL (normal 150,000–400,000)

Pathophysiology

Cellulitis in or near the orbit is due to infection and is divided into two types: **periorbital** (preseptal or preorbital), which is less worrisome and accounts for most cases (roughly **85–90%**), and **orbital** (postseptal), which is more worrisome. Once infection involves the tissue in the orbit proper (i.e., extends **behind the orbital septum** [palpebral fascia]), orbital cellulitis is said to be present. Infections usually reach the orbital region via one of three routes: *internal extension* from sinusitis, *external extension* from a skin wound or insect bite, or *hematogenous spread* (uncommon). Thus, the common etiologic bacteria include sinusitis bugs (e.g., *Haemophilus influenzae, Strepococcus pneumoniae*) and cellulitis bugs (e.g., *Staphylococcus aureus, S. pyogenes*). Most cases occur in the **pediatric age group.**

Diagnosis & Treatment

Historically, patients may have had symptoms of **sinusitis** or a **break in the skin near the eye** (e.g., trauma, insect bite). This is followed by eyelid swelling and redness, which occur in both types of infections, usually accompanied by **fever.** At least 90% of the time, symptoms are *unilateral.*

On exam, **edema and erythema of the eyelids** and surrounding skin are seen. **Conjunctivitis** and/or **nasal discharge** (with sinusitis) are fairly common. Patients generally have fever, and **leukocytosis** may also be present. If the patient has trouble moving the eye (i.e., **ophthalmoplegia,** usually due to pain), **decreased visual acuity, proptosis** (i.e., the eye bulges outward), or **eye pain,** orbital cellulitis is presumed to be present, as these symptoms/signs are characteristically *absent* in periorbital cellulitis.

Treatment is empiric *intravenous antibiotics* on an *inpatient* basis after blood cultures have been obtained. A **second- or third-generation cephalosporin** or **extended-spectrum penicillin** (e.g., ampicillin/sulbactam or piperacillin/tazobactam) are common choices. If orbital cellulitis is suspected clinically, order a **CT scan of the orbits** to exclude an **abscess,** which may require surgical drainage.

More High-Yield Facts

Feared, though fortunately rare complications include **permanent vision loss** and intracranial extension, which may cause **meningitis, cavernous sinus thrombosis,** or an **intracranial abscess.**

Other common eyelid lesions: a **hordeolum** (stye) is a **painful** red lump *near* the lid margin, while a **chalazion** is a **painless** lump *away* from the lid margin. Treat both with *warm compresses*. Incision and drainage may be needed for a chalazion if conservative treatment fails.

Case 12

Orthopedics

History

A 41-year-old man is suffering from low back pain. He says the pain started a few days ago and is fairly constant and dull, with an intensity of 6/10. The patient denies trauma, fever, weight loss, neurologic symptoms, or musculoskeletal pain elsewhere in the body. The pain has not interfered with his sleep; is not worse at any particular time of the day; and is not exacerbated by normal activity. However, it is aggravated by strenuous activity, and he has been "taking it easy" to avoid discomfort. He helped his sister move into her new house a week ago, but his occupation does not involve lifting. The patient does not exercise regularly and smokes 1 pack of cigarettes per day. His past medical history is remarkable for hypertension, for which he takes daily hydrochlorothiazide. He also has been taking aspirin for his back pain, with some relief. Family history is noncontributory. The patient denies alcohol or illicit drug use.

Exam

T: 98.6°F   BP: 136/88   RR: 14/min.   P: 76/min.

The man is obese, but in no acute distress. Head, neck, chest, and abdominal exams are normal. No focal tenderness of the lower back is noted upon palpation, and no masses are appreciated. There is full range of motion at all joints. Muscle strength and tone are normal. No erythema or effusion of the joints in the lower extremities is appreciated. When you raise his legs while he is lying on his back, the back pain is not aggravated. Reflexes are normal and symmetric in the upper and lower extremities; no focal neurologic deficits are apparent; and the remainder of the examination is normal.

Tests

Hemoglobin: 15 g/dL (normal 14–18)   WBCs: 6800/μL (normal 4500–11,000)
Platelets: 270,000/μL   ESR: 8 mm/hr (normal 0–20)
   (normal 150,000–400,000)   Urinalysis: normal
AP and lateral lumbar spine x-rays: see figures

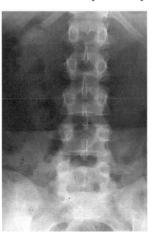
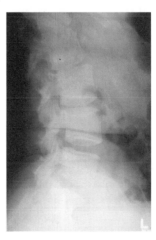

Low back pain (LBP), etiology uncertain

The lumbar spine x-rays are normal.

Pathophysiology

LBP is an extremely common complaint, affecting **up to 70%** of people at some point during their lives. Most cases resolve spontaneously and are **idiopathic,** due to **strain,** or from joint **degeneration.** Sometimes chronic pain develops for unknown reasons. Other etiologies for back pain include **lumbar disc disease, spinal stenosis, trauma, spondylolisthesis, arthritis, autoimmune disorders, neoplasm, infection,** and **etiologies outside the back and spine** (e.g., abdominal aortic aneurysm, peptic ulcer disease). Idiopathic causes are most common and are more likely in those who are **overweight, smoke,** and/or engage in **heavy or repetitive lifting** (e.g., occupational).

Diagnosis & Treatment

Your job is to determine which cases of LBP can be treated conservatively without extensive work-up, and which cases require more aggressive work-up and/or intervention. "Benign" LBP is often **related to recent activity,** is *mild to moderate* in intensity, and *rarely* interferes with sleep to any significant extent. If **fever, weight loss, neurologic symptoms/signs, worsening symptoms over time** with conservative management, and/or **pain that is severe or worse at night** are present, *more extensive investigation is needed.*

In cases without "warning" symptoms, **conservative management** is usually indicated. Initial **lumbar spine x-rays** are commonly obtained, though the diagnostic yield is low, to exclude obvious abnormalities (e.g., fracture, spondylolisthesis, degenerative changes, metastatic disease). Most patients get better *within 2 months,* regardless of the treatment. **NSAIDs** or **acetaminophen** (beware the narcotic-seeker, who may be malingering) are used for symptom relief. Bed rest is *not* usually helpful and should only be advocated for a day or 2 *if at all.* **Stretching and strengthening exercises** may be beneficial.

In the setting of associated worrisome or chronic symptoms, further work-up depends on the suspected etiology. For suspected back pathology, **MRI** of the lumbar spine is generally favored if plain films are negative. **CT scans** are best in the setting of acute trauma. Other tests may include a rheumatoid factor titer and prostate specific antigen (suspected prostate cancer with metastases, a not uncommon presentation).

More High-Yield Facts

Spinal stenosis is a common cause of neurologic leg pain in the elderly. Patients classically describe **increasing leg pain with walking or standing** that is **relieved by sitting, lying down, or leaning forward** (can mimic vascular claudication). Surgery may be helpful if conservative management fails.

Case 13

Orthopedics

History

A 44-year-old woman comes to your office with a chief complaint of intermittent numbness, tingling, and clumsiness in her hands. She says the symptoms began a few months ago and have been getting worse, to the point where they are starting to interfere with her work as a typist. The patient states the symptoms seem to come on intermittently and randomly, and are slightly worse in her dominant right hand. She has strong tingling sensations in both hands, as though her hands have "fallen asleep," and this often wakes her up at night. At times, the patient has dropped items she was holding in her hand due to intermittent "clumsiness." She denies fever, fatigue, weight changes, or other musculoskeletal or neurologic symptoms. Her past medical history is unremarkable. She takes no medications and has not been sexually active in the last few years. The patient denies smoking and drinks alcohol only on special occasions.

Exam

T: 98.8°F   BP: 122/78   RR: 14/min.   P: 76/min.

The patient is fit and healthy appearing. Head, neck, chest, abdomen, and lower extremity exams are normal. She has mild sensory loss in the thumb and first two fingers of both hands. Percussion of the volar aspect of each distal wrist reproduces the patient's typical tingling symptoms. No hypothenar atrophy or weakness is noted in either hand. The remainder of the examination is unremarkable.

Tests

Hemoglobin: 15 g/dL (normal 12–16)
WBCs: 7800/μL (normal 4500–11,000)
Platelets: 280,000/μL (normal 150,000–400,000)
Glucose: 92 mg/dL (normal fasting: 70–110)
Creatinine: 0.9 mg/dL (normal 0.6–1.4)
ESR: 8 mm/hr (normal 0–20)
Thyroid stimulating hormone (TSH): 2.6 μU/mL (normal 0.5–5)
Urinalysis: normal

Carpal tunnel syndrome (CTS)

Pathophysiology

CTS is due to **median nerve compression** at the wrist. The median nerve and the extrinsic finger and thumb flexors go through the carpal tunnel, a narrow canal bound by the carpal bones and the flexor retinaculum. In most cases of CTS, the cause of the compression is either **idiopathic** or due to: (1) a *change in the size of the tunnel* (e.g., carpal fracture/dislocation, osteophyte formation); (2) an *increase in volume of the contents* of the canal (e.g., synovial proliferation or tendon/muscle hypertrophy from repetitive wrist flexion); (3) a *space-occupying lesion* (e.g., canal lipoma or ganglion cyst); or (4) median nerve *neuritis* (e.g., from diabetes). These changes to the tunnel and/or nerve are classically caused by **repetitive forceful wrist flexion,** but may also result from **hypothyroidism, acromegaly, diabetes, pregnancy, arthritis,** and **gout.** *Women are affected more often* than men, and those affected are usually **middle-aged.**

Diagnosis & Treatment

The classic history is **tingling and numbness,** sometimes with **pain,** in the *thumb and first two fingers.* **Hand weakness or clumsiness** is also common, as the median nerve supplies the thenar muscles. Symptoms are most often *unilateral,* but can be bilateral in one-third to one-half of cases. **Nocturnal wakening from hand paresthesias or pain** is classic. There may be a history of repetitive wrist flexion (e.g., occupational or sports-related).

On exam, look for **decreased sensation in the median nerve distribution** (radial aspect of the palm, thumb, and first two fingers). Tapping on the median nerve (i.e., volar aspect of the distal wrist or proximal palm) often causes paresthesias in the median nerve distribution; this is called a positive **Tinel's sign. Phalen's test** involves flexing both wrists and putting the dorsal aspect of the hands against each other with the fingers dependent for 60 seconds. The test is positive if paresthesias/sensory disturbances occur.

Basic lab studies include **TSH, chemistry profile,** and **ESR** to rule out systemic causes. Other causes (e.g., acromegaly) are pursued in select patients. **Electromyography** and **nerve conduction velocity studies** are the gold standard for diagnosis. They are used in equivocal cases, prior to surgery, and for legal reasons (e.g., workers' compensation).

Initial management is *conservative,* with supportive **wrist splints** and **NSAIDs.** Corticosteroid injections can also help relieve symptoms. Surgery (carpal tunnel release) is employed only for those who fail conservative management.

More High-Yield Facts

Nerve conduction velocity is *slowed* if CTS is present.

Case 14

Orthopedics

History

A 5-year-old boy is brought to your office by his mother for left knee pain and swelling. The mother thinks the symptoms started about 1 week ago when the child bumped his knee after a fall. She says he has not had a fever, skin laceration, or pain or swelling in other areas. The child is otherwise in good health and has no significant past medical history. Vaccinations are up-to-date, and the mother says her son is intelligent and well adjusted. He takes no regular medications, though she has been giving him acetaminophen for pain the last few days. Family history is noncontributory.

Exam

T: 99.2°F   BP: 90/62   RR: 18/min.   P: 88/min.

The child appears well developed and well nourished. Height and weight are appropriate for age. When you ask him to walk, he favors the right leg and has a slight limp. There is increased warmth above the left knee and an underlying palpable, firm mass. The knee joint itself does not seem to be involved, and no joint effusion is evident. Passive range of motion (ROM) at both knees and hips is normal, though ROM is reduced in the left knee secondary to pain. Reflexes are normal and symmetric; there are no focal neurologic deficits or skin findings; and the remainder of the exam is unremarkable.

Tests

Hemoglobin: 11 g/dL (normal 11–13)   WBCs: 9800/μL (normal 5000–15,000)
Platelets: 360,000/μL   X-rays of left knee: see figures
  (normal 150,000–400,000)

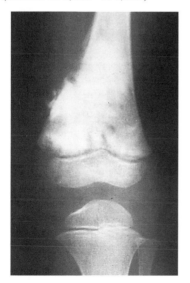 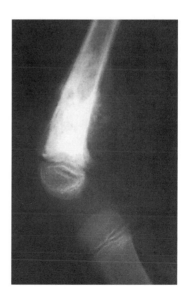

Osteogenic sarcoma

The x-rays reveal an aggressive lesion in the distal metaphysis of the femur, with bone destruction and extension into the adjacent soft tissues. The classic **Codman's triangle**-type periosteal reaction is seen proximally.

Pathophysiology

Osteogenic sarcoma is the **most common primary bone malignancy** (excluding *multiple myeloma*) and is usually seen in patients under age 30, classically in those **10–25 years old.** Most cases are idiopathic, though in older adults the malignancy may be related to **previous radiation** or **Paget's disease.** Seventy-five percent of cases occur in the **long bones,** and half occur around the knee (i.e., **distal femur** or **proximal tibia**).

Diagnosis & Treatment

The classic history is **pain** about the knee in an adolescent, often for weeks or months, though a history of recent trauma is often given. **Limping** and pain that is **worse at night** are also classic. **Intermittent fever** may occur. Systemic symptoms from metastasis, *most commonly to the lungs,* is unusual at presentation.

Exam may be normal, but a **palpable mass** is present in more than half of cases, often associated with **local warmth.** Radiographs will lead you to suspect the diagnosis. Osteogenic sarcomas generally arise from the **metaphysis,** usually around the knee, and **destroy bone** as well as produce osteoid matrix (**calcified, cloud-like pattern on x-ray,** as in this case). **Periosteal reaction** with new bone formation is classic, often in the pattern of **Codman's triangle** (periosteum is elevated and forms a triangular shape), or a **"sunburst/sunray"** pattern (spicules of bone radiate in multiple directions like the rays of the sun). The diagnosis is confirmed with **biopsy.**

Treatment includes **chemotherapy and surgical resection,** which may require amputation. If the tumor can be completely resected, 5-year survival is about **70–80%.**

More High-Yield Facts

Ewing's sarcoma is the other common primary bone malignancy in children, classically affecting those **aged 5–15 years old.** The lesion usually occurs in the **diaphysis** (mid-portion of a long bone) and may cause an **"onion-skin"** type of periosteal reaction (multiple layers of reactive peiosteal new bone formation). Treatment is chemotherapy and surgery.

Roughly 95% of bone malignancies are **metastatic;** only 5% are primary tumors.

Case 15

Orthopedics

History

A 22-year-old man presents to the emergency department 6 hours after sustaining a knee injury in a basketball game. The patient claims he went up for a rebound and when he came down he heard a "pop," and immediately felt his knee "give way." His knee swelled up quickly, and he has been unable to bear weight on it since the injury. The patient is otherwise in good health and denies similar symptoms in the past. Past medical history is unremarkable, and he takes no medications. He smokes and drinks alcohol "on occasion," and is sexually active with his girlfriend of 2 years. Family history is noncontributory.

Exam

T: 98.4°F   BP: 122/74   RR: 14/min.   P: 88/min.

The patient is healthy appearing, but has significant pain. His left knee is swollen with an obvious effusion, and he is unable to bear significant weight on it. Range of motion in this knee is guarded, painful, and limited. With the patient's hips flexed at 45 degrees and knees in 90 degrees of flexion, you ask him to relax. After stabilizing his left femur, you grip the back of his upper calf and pull the proximal left tibia gently forward, repeating this procedure on the right. There is asymmetry between the two sides during this maneuver, with a greater anterior movement of the tibia in relation to the femur on the left side.

Tests

Hemoglobin: 15 g/dL (normal 14–18)
WBCs: 8800/μL (normal 4500–11,000)
Platelets: 340,000/μL (normal 150,000–400,000)
X-rays of the left knee: effusion without an identifiable fracture
Arthrocentesis: grossly bloody fluid

Pathophysiology

The ACL helps to *prevent excessive anterior movement of the tibia* in relation to the femur and also provides some resistance to varus and valgus stress on the knee. It is the **most commonly injured knee ligament,** and is usually torn by **hyperextension** of the knee or an excessive **valgus force** (from lateral to medial) on the knee (as in a "clipping" injury in football). A *direct blow* to the front of a flexed knee (e.g., a dashboard injury) or *sudden deceleration or twisting* while running can also cause ACL injury. With ACL disruption, the knee joint becomes unstable.

Diagnosis & Treatment

The classic history involves a mechanism of injury as described above, and sudden onset of knee pain. Patients classically hear a **"pop"** and claim that the knee **"buckled," "gave way," "locked up," or "popped out"** at the time of injury. **Swelling** develops *immediately* after the injury, and **range of motion** (ROM) **is painful and limited.** Patients are usually **unable to walk or bear significant weight** on the knee.

On exam, a positive **anterior drawer test** is classic (as in this case). A **joint effusion** generally is present—typically due to **hemarthrosis** (roughly 70% of patients with an acute knee injury and hemarthrosis have an ACL tear). ROM is restricted and painful. X-rays are generally *negative* for fracture, but usually demonstrate a **joint effusion. MRI** is often obtained when surgery is contemplated, and can demonstrate the tear and other associated injuries.

Treatment depends on the patient's situation, and may include **conservative management** (physical therapy, etc.) or **surgical reconstruction** of the ACL. Younger patients and athletes are often advised to have surgery.

More High-Yield Facts

Posterior cruciate ligament injuries result in a positive **posterior drawer test** (can push tibia backward more than usual with the knee in 90° of flexion). **Medial collateral ligament** (MCL) injuries commonly coexist with ACL injuries and result in a positive **abduction (valgus) stress test** (an abnormal degree of *abduction* of the knee joint, demonstrated by holding the knee still at 30° of flexion and *abducting* the ankle). **Lateral collateral ligament** injuries result in a positive **adduction (varus) stress test** (abnormal *adduction* of the knee joint, demonstrated by holding the knee still at 30° of flexion and *adducting* the ankle).

The **unhappy triad** knee injury is damage to the ACL, MCL and medial meniscus, which classically occurs after a "clipping" injury in football.

Case 16

Orthopedics

History

A 74-year-old woman is seeking emergency attention for left hip pain after a fall in her home that occurred a few hours ago. She was feeling well up until the fall, and did not lose consciousness. She is unable to bear significant weight on her left leg due to the pain. Past medical history is significant for severe chronic obstructive pulmonary disease that has been frequently treated with courses of corticosteroids. The patient also regularly uses four different metered-dose inhalers: albuterol, ipratropium, beclomethasone, and salmeterol. She has a 50 pack-year smoking history, drinks alcohol on a daily basis, and is physically inactive. Family history is noncontributory.

Exam

T: 98.8°F   BP: 140/88   RR: 16/min.   P: 90/min.

The patient has a slight, thin build and is clearly in pain. She holds her left leg in such a way that her thigh is externally rotated and abducted to reduce her discomfort. There is a slight leg length discrepancy, with the left leg slightly shorter than the right. The patient resists both active and passive motion at the hip due to pain. No focal neurologic deficits are evident. Pulses are symmetric and normal in the lower extremities. The remainder of the exam is unremarkable.

Tests

Hemoglobin: 13 g/dL (normal 12–16)
WBCs: 8400/μL (normal 4500–11,000)
Platelets: 320,000/μL (normal 150,000–400,000)
Left hip x-ray: see figure

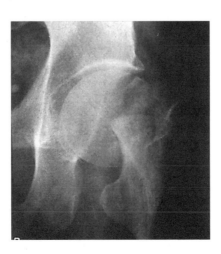

Hip fracture

The x-ray shows a left femoral neck (hip) fracture, with some overlap of the femoral head and neck.

Pathophysiology

The great majority of hip fractures, which usually are *femoral neck* fractures, are seen in those **over age 70.** More than 90% are associated with a fall. Other than age, one of the primary risk factors is **osteoporosis,** which weakens the bones and increases the risk of fracture (fractures can occur after minor trauma, e.g., a fall in the home). After an osteoporotic hip fracture, there is at least a 15% excessive mortality rate, and less than one-third of patients will have returned to their previous level of functioning 1 year later. Therefore, osteoporosis is a major health problem. In young adults, hip fractures are associated with high-energy trauma, such as **motor vehicle accidents.**

Diagnosis & Treatment

The classic patient is an **elderly white or Asian female** with other osteoporosis risk factors (e.g., **smoking/alcohol abuse, thin body habitus, poor calcium intake, family history, corticosteroid use, sedentary lifestyle**) who falls and presents with hip pain.

On exam, patients classically hold their thigh in **external rotation** and **abduction** to reduce discomfort. Slight **shortening of the affected extremity** may be present. Generalized pain of the hip or **groin pain referred down the medial thigh** is typical, and hip motion is limited. Patients generally refuse to bear weight or walk with a limp that favors the unaffected side. X-rays typically reveal a fracture. If a fracture is not seen but is suspected clinically, order **follow-up films in 1–2 weeks or an MRI** of the hip.

Treatment depends on the patient, but generally includes **open or closed reduction,** or **hip arthroplasty.** Hip arthroplasty (i.e., artificial hip replacement) is generally favored for patients older than 70. Classic complications of hip fractures include **avascular necrosis, deep venous thrombosis/pulmonary embolus,** and **infection.**

More High-Yield Facts

Stress fractures of the hip are uncommon, but classically occur in **long-distance runners** and cause vague hip pain made *worse* by activity. A plain x-ray or bone scan generally allows the diagnosis. Patients should temporarily *avoid* strenuous activity and excessive weight bearing until the pain resolves, or they risk progression to a complete fracture.

Avascular necrosis of the hip (i.e., femoral head) can be associated with fracture, **corticosteroid** use, **sickle cell disease, alcoholism,** and **lupus,** or it can be idiopathic (e.g., **Legg-Calvé-Perthes disease**).

Orthopedics

History

A 31-year-old man has come to the emergency department because of a right shoulder injury sustained during a pick-up football game. The patient claims he was trying to make a tackle with his outstretched right arm as an opponent ran by him. He immediately experienced pain and felt his arm "go dead." The patient says his arm movement is now limited secondary to pain. The pain is somewhat relieved when he holds his right arm up with his left hand. He was previously healthy and has no significant past medical history. He takes no medications and has not had a similar injury in the past.

Exam

T: 98.6°F   BP: 130/78   RR: 14/min.   P: 80/min.

The patient is athletic appearing and in no acute distress. On visual inspection, there is asymmetry between the shoulders, with a loss of the normal, rounded contour of the right shoulder, which appears somewhat square. The right humeral head is palpable through the axilla. The patient cannot fully abduct or internally rotate his right arm, and is unable to touch his left shoulder with his right hand. No focal neurologic deficits are evident, and distal pulses in the upper extremities are normal and symmetric. The remainder of the examination is unremarkable.

Tests

Right shoulder x-ray: see figure

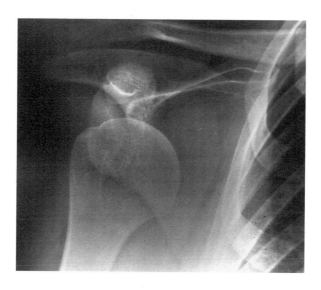

Shoulder dislocation

The x-ray shows the humeral head situated inferior and medial to the glenoid, which is characteristic of an anterior dislocation.

Pathophysiology

Shoulder (i.e., humeral head) dislocations are generally either **anterior (90–95%** of cases) or **posterior** in relation to the glenoid. Anterior dislocations are usually due to a force that causes *external rotation and/or hyperextension* of an arm that is already abducted, externally rotated, and/or extended. **Recurrence is common** (roughly one-third to one-half of adolescents and young adults after initial dislocation) due to associated shoulder joint instability. Posterior dislocations are rare, classically due to **seizures or electrocution,** and may be **bilateral.**

Diagnosis & Treatment

The classic history includes a typical mechanism of injury, immediate **pain,** a feeling of the arm **"going dead,"** and a markedly **reduced range of motion** (ROM). Patients often notice an obvious shoulder contour deformity and may reduce pain by **elevating the affected arm with the opposite hand.**

On exam, the affected shoulder **loses its normal rounded contour** and appears **square.** The humeral head is abnormally palpable, and "emptiness" in the glenoid fossa (where the humeral head is supposed to be) can be appreciated. Patients *cannot* fully internally rotate or abduct the arm and are *unable* to touch the unaffected shoulder with the hand of the affected side. Though uncommon, **axillary nerve injury** can occur with a dislocation (watch for deltoid paralysis and absent sensation on the lateral shoulder). X-rays confirm the diagnosis and should be assessed for associated fractures.

Treatment is prompt **closed reduction,** performed in any of a number of ways (e.g., gentle longitudinal traction on the arm with countertraction to the torso, or lying the patient prone on a table and tying a weight to the wrist as it hangs over the side). Give **pain medication** *prior* to reduction, and obtain an x-ray afterwards to confirm reduction. Also, perform a full **neurologic and vascular exam** of the arm *both before and after* reduction. After reduction, the patient is typically kept in a **splint** until pain improves **(1–3 weeks),** and then physical rehabilitation to restore ROM and strengthen the shoulder girdle muscles begins. Those with **recurrent dislocations** generally benefit from **surgery** to stabilize the shoulder joint.

More High-Yield Facts

The **rotator cuff** includes the *supraspinatus, infraspinatus, subscapularis,* and *teres minor* muscles. A "torn rotator cuff" most commonly refers to a tear in the **supraspinatus** tendon.

Case 18

Orthopedics

History

You are called to the nursery to perform a newborn exam on a child delivered an hour ago. This is the mother's first baby, and the delivery was via cesarean section at term due to a breech presentation. Family history is unremarkable and APGAR scores were 8 and 9 at one and five minutes, respectively. The mother received regular prenatal care, has no medical problems, and did not smoke, drink alcohol, or use other drugs during the pregnancy.

Exam

Vital signs: normal

Head, neck, chest, and abdominal exams are normal. No neurologic deficits are appreciated. You note asymmetry between the fat folds of the child's thighs. While she is laying on her back, you flex both her hips and knees while the hips are adducted. When you subsequently apply gentle downward pressure on the knees, a palpable "clunk" is felt on the right. You then abduct the hips with the knees and hips still flexed, which again results in a palpable clunk on the right. The remainder of the examination is unremarkable.

Tests

Hemoglobin: 19 g/dL (normal 17–22)
Total bilirubin: 1.1 mg/dL (normal < 6)

Pathophysiology

CHD refers to a spectrum of conditions that result in **inadequate development** of hip structures, which can range from mild abnormalities in the shape of the acetabulum to frank dislocation and instability of the hip. Roughly **1%** of children in the newborn nursery have dislocatable hips. The classic risk factors for CHD include being a **first child, female sex, breech delivery, oligohydramnios,** and **family history.** It has been theorized that the maternal hormones **estrogen** and **relaxin** contribute to CHD.

Diagnosis & Treatment

Though it can present later, CHD is classically discovered in a **newborn** being examined routinely in the nursery. Historical risk factors discussed above may or may not be present.

On exam, any of three classic findings may be present: **(1) asymmetry of the fat folds in the thigh** may be seen due to apparent shortening of the leg from dislocation. An adjunct to this finding is known as the **Galeazzi sign:** with the child on his or her back, the legs held together, the hips and knees flexed to 90°, and the soles of the feet pressed flat against the examining table, different knee height may be seen due to the apparent thigh length discrepancy with a unilateral dislocation. **(2)** The **Barlow test** attempts to passively dislocate the hip. With the knees and hips flexed to 90° and the infant lying on his or her back, a gentle downward (i.e., posterior) force is exerted on the femur. A **palpable clunk** indicates hip dislocation. **(3)** The **Ortolani manuever,** which can reduce a dislocated hip, is also performed. In the same position, with the knees and hips flexed to 90°, the hip is abducted. A **palpable or audible clunk** (*not* a high-pitched click, which is a *normal* finding) indicates reduction of a dislocated hip. After 3 months of age, the Barlow and Ortolani signs are *unreliable* and **limited hip abduction** is the main finding.

If the physical exam is suspicious, an **ultrasound** of the hip is the preferred test to confirm the diagnosis, as the unossified cartilage of the hip structures allows better visualization than x-ray **before 3–5 months of age.** Plain x-rays are used after this age. Initial treatment is with a **Pavlik harness,** which helps to hold the hips in a somewhat *flexed and abducted* position to maintain stability of the joint while development proceeds. **Casting** or (rarely) surgery may be needed if conservative management fails.

More High-Yield Facts

Bowlegs (genu varum) and **knock knees (genu valgum)** are most often mild and typically resolve spontaneously by mid-childhood.

Case 19

Orthopedics

History

A 12-year-old boy is brought in by his father for right knee pain that began 2 weeks ago after a fall. Upon questioning, the child admits to mild knee pain that had been present prior to the fall. The father has noticed his son limping since the injury, and brought him in when he saw no improvement. The patient is otherwise healthy and has no significant past medical history, other than obesity. He denies other musculoskeletal symptoms, takes no medications, and is not sexually active.

Exam

T: 98.8°F   BP: 110/68   RR: 14/min.   P: 82/min.

The patient is obese and in no acute distress. When asked to walk, he demonstrates a slight limp that favors the left leg. The right knee has a normal appearance, with no erythema, effusion, or increased warmth apparent. The knee also has full active and passive range of motion (ROM). During examination of the hip, pain results from passive ROM, with limited internal rotation and abduction. Hip flexion produces marked pain and causes the child to rotate the hip externally. No neurologic or pulse abnormalities are noted in the right leg. The remainder of the examination is unremarkable.

Tests

Hemoglobin: 13 g/dL (normal 11–13)
Platelets: 240,000/μL
   (normal 150,000–400,000)
Knee x-rays: normal

WBCs: 7800/μL (normal 4500–13,000)
C-reactive protein: 0.3 mg/dL
   (normal 0–0.8)
Pelvic x-ray: see figure

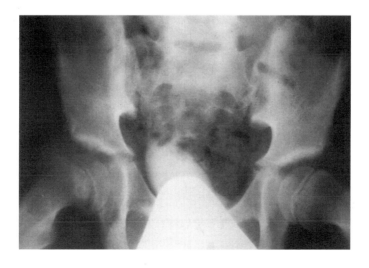

Slipped capital femoral epiphysis (SCFE)

The x-ray shows the right femoral epiphysis displaced medially relative to the femoral shaft.

Pathophysiology

SCFE describes "slippage" of the epiphysis of the femoral head (i.e., the *capital femoral epiphysis*) off the remainder of the femur, and can range from mild to severe. The femoral epiphysis becomes **displaced medially and posteriorly** relative to the femoral shaft. SCFE is **idiopathic,** affects **boys twice as often** as girls, and tends to occur during the *adolescent growth spurt* (**ages 9–15**) in those who are **obese.**

Diagnosis & Treatment

Patients are classically **overweight adolescent males** with an insidious onset of **pain in the hip, groin, thigh, or knee,** which often causes a **limp.** A classic history is initial pain that is intermittent and gradual in onset, often with sudden worsening after a recent trauma.

On exam, there is typically mild to severe pain on motion of the hip with **limited internal rotation and abduction.** Flexion of the hip causes pain and **obligatory external rotation of the thigh.** If pain is referred to the knee, examination will reveal no knee abnormalities or limitation of movement. *Any knee pain in a child should prompt evaluation of the hip as well as the knee on the affected side.* The diagnosis is confirmed with a **pelvic x-ray,** which allows a comparison between the two hips so that subtle cases are more easily detected.

Treatment is prompt **surgical pinning** to fix the femoral epiphysis to the femoral shaft, preventing further slippage.

More High-Yield Facts

Legg-Calvé-Perthes (LCP) disease, the "other" common childhood hip disorder, involves idiopathic **osteonecrosis** (i.e., avascular necrosis) of the proximal femoral epiphysis (affects the same area as SCFE). It typically occurs in **5- to 8-year-olds** (helping differentiate it clinically from SCFE) and is **three to five times more common in boys.** Symptoms and physical exam are similar to those in SCFE, but patients are usually *not* overweight.

In LCP, the x-ray may show patchy sclerotic densities in, and an irregular surface of, the proximal femoral epiphysis, or there may be **fragmentation or collapse** of the epiphysis (depends on the stage—you would likely be shown a fragmented or collapsed epiphysis). The condition is **bilateral** in up to 20% of cases. Initial treatment is **conservative,** with ROM exercises and **leg braces.** Surgery is employed if conservative management fails.

Orthopedics

History

A 59-year-old man comes to the emergency department with the chief complaint of a red, swollen left toe. The patient denies pain and says his symptoms began a few weeks ago, but he has been reluctant to see his doctor. He recalls no history of trauma. He is a type II diabetic, and mentions that his blood sugar has been high lately even though he has been following his diet and taking his medications as prescribed. Past medical history is also remarkable for hypertension and stable angina. The patient's medications include lisinopril, metformin, troglitazone, acarbose, hydrochlorothiazide, and as-needed nitroglycerin. He has a long smoking history, but does not drink alcohol and is not currently sexually active.

Exam

T: 101.9°F   BP: 144/98   RR: 16/min.   P: 94/min.

The man, though obese, is not in acute distress. Head, neck, and chest examinations are unremarkable, except for changes in the retinas consistent with nonproliferative diabetic retinopathy. The left great toe is markedly erythematous, hot, and swollen, and on the underside you note a foul-smelling, purulent discharge that can be expressed from a small opening in the skin. The toe is not tender to palpation or manipulation. In fact, the patient has markedly decreased vibratory sense and two-point discrimination in both feet below the level of the ankle. The remainder of the examination is unremarkable.

Tests

Hemoglobin: 14 g/dL (normal 12–16)
WBCs: 16,800/µL (normal 4500–11,000)
Platelets: 340,000/µL
    (normal 150,000–400,000)
Glucose: 284 mg/dL
    (normal fasting 70–110)
Creatinine: 1.2 mg/dL
    (normal 0.6–1.5 mg/dL)
BUN: 35 mg/dL (normal 8–25)
Uric acid: 3.8 mg/dL (normal 3–7)
Left foot x-ray: see figure

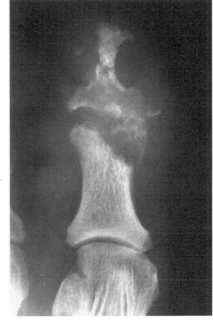

Osteomyelitis

The x-ray shows prominent bony destruction of the proximal and distal phalanges of the great toe, with associated soft tissue swelling.

Pathophysiology

Though the "diabetic foot" is a classic clinical scenario for osteomyelitis, there are other ways it can develop. Most infections are **bacterial,** and organisms can reach the bone via three routes: *hematogenous* (common in children and IV drug abusers), *spread from adjacent soft tissue* (e.g., foot ulcer, sinusitis), or *direct inoculation* (e.g., open fractures, penetrating trauma, or surgical bone procedures). The most common organism is *Staphylococcus aureus,* but *Salmonella* is the classic organism in sickle cell patients, and most diabetic foot infections with osteomyelitis are **polymicrobial.**

Diagnosis & Treatment

Patients usually have prominent risk factors for osteomyelitis, such as **diabetes, neuropathy, arterial insufficiency, sickle cell disease, trauma with disruption of the skin, bone surgery,** or **IV drug abuse.** In the absence of neuropathy, **pain** is almost universally present, and a history of **fever** is common.

On exam, there is generally **tenderness** over the area of infected bone, along with **erythema, edema, and/or increased temperature** of the overlying skin. **Draining pus** in this setting almost clinches the diagnosis. Fever, leukocytosis, and an elevated ESR are typical. The changes of osteomyelitis—usually **bony destruction**—take **1–2 weeks for x-ray visibility.** If x-rays are negative but osteomyelitis is still suspected, order a **"triple-phase" bone scan,** which is more sensitive and becomes positive earlier than x-rays.

The treatment is **antibiotics,** which are generally withheld until blood cultures and needle aspiration of the bone or bone biopsy are performed. Aspiration of an adjacent abscess or arthrocentesis of an affected joint may also be helpful, depending on the setting. Note that swabbing in or around affected skin overlying the bone (i.e., draining pus or a foot ulcer) is usually *not helpful,* as skin flora make the results of these culture methods *unreliable.* Empiric, **broad-spectrum IV antibiotics** (e.g., nafcillin) to cover common potential bugs such as *S. aureus* are started while awaiting culture results. Treatment usually takes **4–8 weeks.**

More High-Yield Facts

Chronic osteomyelitis is difficult to treat and may result in a **sequestrum** (dead bone that acts as a reservoir for reinfection) or a bone abscess (i.e., **Brodie's abscess**). Surgical **debridement** and other aggressive measures (e.g., bone grafting) are often needed in this setting.

Orthopedics

History

A 47-year-old man complains of lower back pain that radiates down the back of his left leg. He says he has had intermittent bouts of this pain in the past, but recently "twisted" his back while lifting a heavy box at home and now has nearly constant pain. He has also noticed some tingling and numbness in the lateral aspect of his foot since the pain became more constant. Lying still in bed often relieves the pain, but he is unable to lie down at work. The patient denies fever, weight loss, pain in other areas, or other neurologic symptoms. Past medical history is otherwise unremarkable, and the only medication he takes is acetaminophen for his back pain. Family and social history are noncontributory.

Exam

T: 98.9°F   BP: 124/80   RR: 14/min.   P: 84/min.

The patient is slightly overweight and appears moderately uncomfortable due to his pain. Head, neck, chest, and abdominal exams are normal. No focal tenderness is present over the back or left leg, though you note some mild muscle spasm in the lower left back. With the patient lying flat on his back, you lift his left heel off the examining table, keeping his left knee straight. This causes "shooting" pains down the back of his left leg. You also note a markedly decreased left ankle jerk and some mild weakness of plantar flexion of the left foot when compared to the right. Decreased sensation over the lateral left foot is also apparent. No other neurologic deficits are appreciated. The remainder of the examination is unremarkable.

Tests

Hemoglobin: 14 g/dL (normal 12–16)
WBCs: 7500/μL (normal 4500–11,000)
Platelets: 230,000/μL (normal 150,000–400,000)
Uric acid: 4.1 mg/dL (normal 3–7)
ESR: 9 mm/hr (normal 0–20)
MRI of the lumbar spine: see figure

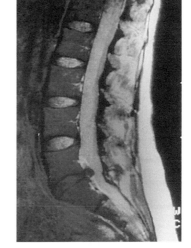

Lumbar disc disease affecting the left S1 nerve root

The MRI shows **herniation** of the L5-S1 disc posterior to the vertebral bodies.

Pathophysiology

Intervertebral disc disease is a common cause of back and neck pain, but rarely results in thoracic spine symptoms. The exact etiology is unknown, but it is presumed to be **degenerative** in origin, as a large percentage of individuals over age 30 (most of whom are asymptomatic) have "bulging" discs on imaging studies. When a disc *herniates,* the central **nucleus pulposus** is squeezed through a tear in its surrounding **annulus fibrosus** like toothpaste out of a tube, usually in a posterolateral direction (though other directions can occur). The lower lumbar spine (L5-S1 and L4-L5 discs) is the most common location. Posterolateral disc herniations irritate the *next lower ipsilateral nerve root* (e.g., a herniated L4-L5 disc affects the L5 nerve root). This can cause neurologic symptoms (i.e., **radiculopathy**).

Diagnosis & Treatment

Intervertebral disc disease can cause vague neck or back pain, but the classic symptom is **pain radiating into an extremity. Sciatica,** or pain radiating to the leg, is often described as a "*shooting*" or "*electrical*" pain.

On exam, the classic finding is a **positive straight-leg raise test** (as described in this case). To be considered positive, this maneuver should *reproduce the sciatica, not just the lower back pain.* Spasm of the back muscles may or may not be present due to local irritation. When the L5-S1 disc is affected, the pain often radiates down into the calf, and a **decreased ankle jerk** reflex, **numbness in the lateral foot,** and/or weakness of the plantarflexors of the foot may be present. An L4-L5 herniation usually affects the L5 nerve root, classically causing **weakness of the foot extensors** and **sensation changes in the medial foot.** The C6-C7 disc is the most commonly affected cervical disc, usually causing C7 nerve root irritation. This can **weaken** and cause a **decreased reflex in the triceps muscle.**

Choose **conservative management** (e.g., analgesics, reduced activity followed by physical therapy/exercise) initially on the boards for suspected disc disease with mild to moderate symptoms, as this works in roughly 85–90% of patients. With **persistent neurologic deficits,** especially when *severe or progressive,* employ **MRI** to identify potentially correctable lesions (e.g., a herniated disc in a location consistent with clinical findings).

More High-Yield Facts

Rarely, a large, midline, lumbar disc herniation causes **cauda equina syndrome.** This occurs when multiple nerve roots are affected by a disc. Look for bilateral leg symptoms, urinary retention, and back pain. MRI is typically used to confirm the diagnosis and treatment is **prompt surgery.**

Urology

History

A 63-year-old man presents to your office with a chief complaint of left flank pain and fever. He says he has been having intermittent fevers and a dull pain in his left flank for the past several weeks. He denies dysuria, but finally decided to come in to see you when he noticed blood in his urine yesterday. The patient mentions that his pants seem loose, which he attributes to weight loss secondary to a decreased appetite. Past medical history is remarkable only for osteoarthritis of both knees, for which he takes acetaminophen. Social history is significant for a 40 pack-year smoking history. Family history is noncontributory.

Exam

T: 100.1°F   BP: 140/88   RR: 14/min.   P: 82/min.

Head, neck, and chest examinations are unremarkable. Abdominal exam reveals no masses and normal bowel sounds. No abdominal or costovertebral angle tenderness is present. Rectal exam is normal. No neurologic, dermatologic, or other abnormalities are appreciated.

Tests

Hemoglobin: 10 g/dL (normal 12–16)
WBCs: 7000/μL (normal 4500–11,000)
Platelets: 430,000/μL (normal 150,000–400,000)
Amylase: 64 U/L (normal 53–123)
AST: 9 U/L (normal 7–27)
Creatinine: 1 mg/dL (normal 0.6–1.5)
BUN: 11 mg/dL (normal 8–25)
Urinalysis: 4+ red blood cells; no protein, bacteria, WBCs, or casts
Abdominal CT scan: see figure

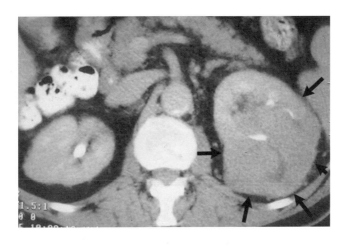

Renal cell carcinoma (RCC)

The CT scan reveals a large soft tissue mass in the left kidney (*arrows*), which is deforming the collecting system.

Pathophysiology

RCC is the *most common primary renal malignancy* (roughly 85% of cases) and most often occurs in those who are **50 to 70 years old.** It is an adenocarcinoma that arises from renal tubular epithelium and is *twice as common in men.* The primary risk factor for RCC is **smoking,** though an increased risk is also seen with **long-term hemodialysis** and **von Hippel-Lindau disease.**

Diagnosis & Treatment

With the advent of modern imaging, most RCC (60%) is *discovered incidentally* when imaging is performed for another reason. The classic symptom triad is **hematuria, flank pain,** and a **palpable mass,** but this combination is present in only 10–15% of patients and indicates advanced disease. **Hematuria,** which is more often microscopic than gross, is the most common presenting symptom. Constitutional symptoms, such as **fever, weight loss, loss of appetite,** and **fatigue,** are fairly common. Patients may also have metastases at initial presentation (approximately 25% of cases), often to the *lungs* (may cause respiratory complaints) or *bones* (bone pain).

On exam, findings are usually minimal, though a flank mass is occasionally palpable, and fever may be present. **Anemia** (25–50% of patients) or, rarely, **erythrocytosis** (due to excess erythropoietin production by the tumor) may be seen. On urinalysis, hematuria is classically present. **Hypertension** or **hypercalcemia,** though rare, also may be seen. In the setting of unexplainable hematuria, order cystoscopy, a CT scan, or intravenous pyelography (IVP) to search for any tumor. Once a suspicious-looking renal mass is discovered, a CT scan of the abdomen and a CT scan of the chest or chest x-ray are used for staging purposes. A bone scan is often ordered in the setting of elevated alkaline phosphatase or bone pain. *Surgical removal* of a suspicious mass is generally *preferred* over a percutaneous renal biopsy.

Surgery offers the best hope for cure, with or without chemotherapy (**interleukin-2** has shown more promise than traditional agents). Invasion of the tumor into the renal vein and inferior vena cava is not uncommon and *does not* preclude surgery, but distant metastases does.

More High-Yield Facts

Persistent (more than one visit), unexplained hematuria *requires further investigation to rule out a urinary tract malignancy,* especially in an adult. Cystoscopy and a CT scan, renal ultrasound, or IVP are usually performed.

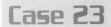

Case 23

Urology

History

A mother brings in her 2-month-old son for a routine well-baby visit. She is concerned because he seems to have only one testicle, and she wonders if he "is deformed." The child has been healthy and has no other problems. The child's growth and development have been on par with the woman's other three children. He was born via vaginal delivery after 33 weeks gestation. There were no problems during the pregnancy, delivery, or neonatal period. Family history is noncontributory.

Exam

Vital signs: normal

The child is alert and active. His length, weight, and head circumference are appropriate for age. Head, neck, and chest examinations are unremarkable. Abdominal exam reveals no masses, tenderness, or organomegaly, and bowel sounds are normal. Rectal exam is also normal. Genitourinary exam reveals only one testicle in the scrotum. In the region of the left inguinal canal, you palpate a testicular-sized, round, soft tissue mass. The penis is unremarkable in appearance. No neurologic, dermatologic, or other abnormalities are appreciated. What should you do to manage this child's condition?

Tests

Hemoglobin: 13 g/dL (normal 11–15)
WBCs: 8000/μL (normal 6000–17,000)
Platelets: 230,000/μL (normal 150,000–400,000)

Undescended testicle, also called cryptorchidism

Pathophysiology

The testicles originate in the abdomen and normally descend *in utero,* reaching the scrotum by the end of the third trimester. At birth, roughly **3% of term infants and 30% of premature infants** have at least one testicle that has failed to reach a normal position within the scrotum. The exact etiology is uncertain, but **hormonal factors** are thought to play a role. The undescended testicle can be located anywhere **along the normal course of testicular descent,** from an intra-abdominal location to the **inguinal canal,** the most common location.

Diagnosis & Treatment

The presence of only one testicle in the scrotum is often due to cryptorchidism. **Congenital absence** of a testicle or an **intersex state** are other, less common etiologies for this finding, which is noticed during the newborn exam. The undescended testicle is typically **palpable in the inguinal canal,** but others are intra-abdominal in location.

There are two primary concerns in those with cryptorchidism: **malignancy** and **infertility.** Other concerns with an undescended testicle are **torsion** and an increased risk of **inguinal hernias** and other genitourinary malformations (e.g., **hypospadias**).

Initial management is **observation,** as roughly 75% of undescended testicles in term infants and 95% in premature infants **descend on their own,** usually within the **first 3 months of life.** By **1 year** of age, an undescended testicle is **very unlikely to descend** on its own, and further treatment is needed. If the testicle is not palpable, imaging (ultrasound or CT scan) can be used to locate it; **laparoscopy** is the gold standard if imaging fails.

Hormonal therapy with **HCG** injections to cause descent can be tried initially, but **surgical orchiopexy** is the most common treatment. The **risk of malignancy** is roughly *10 times higher* in an undescended testicle (usually a seminoma), and orchiopexy, though it does *not* reduce the risk of malignancy, facilitates testicular examination. **Orchiectomy** is used for abnormal-appearing intra-abdominal testicles. *Fertility is reduced* regardless of treatment, but advocates believe earlier surgical intervention increases fertility rates. The **opposite testicle,** even if descended, **is also abnormal** and has an increased risk of malignancy and decreased sperm production.

More High-Yield Facts

A **retractile testis** is a *normal finding that requires no treatment.* The testicle is sometimes found within the scrotum (e.g., during a warm bath), but often retracts up out of the scrotum due to an active cremasteric reflex.

Case 24

Urology

History

A 53-year-old woman is troubled by dysuria, frequent urination, and chronic low back pain. She has a history of urinary tract infections and believes she has another one. The previous infections were treated successfully with antibiotics. She says that a few months ago she was treated on an inpatient basis with intravenous antibiotics, because the infection "went all the way up to my kidney." The patient has no other significant past medical history and is not currently taking any medications. She does not smoke or drink alcohol, and has no known anatomic urinary tract abnormalities.

Exam

T: 99.8°F   BP: 130/84   RR: 16/min.   P: 82/min.

The woman is thin and in no acute distress. Head, neck, and chest exams are normal. Abdominal exam reveals normal bowel sounds and no abdominal tenderness or masses. There is mild costovertebral tenderness bilaterally. Rectal, genital, neurologic, and dermatologic exams are unremarkable.

Tests

Hemoglobin: 14 g/dL (normal 12 -16)
WBCs: 14,100/μL (normal 4500–11,000)
Platelets: 340,000/μL
  (normal 150,000–400,000)
Creatinine: 1.4 mg/dL (normal 0.6–1.5)
BUN: 21 mg/dL (normal 8–25)
Urinalysis: pH 8, 3+ WBC, 4+ RBC, 4+ bacteria, nitrite positive, 3+ leukocyte esterase
Plain abdominal radiograph: see figure

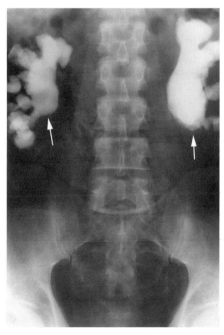

Bilateral **staghorn** renal calculi with urinary tract infection

The x-ray shows large, radiopaque calculi (*arrows*) filling the renal pelvis and calyces.

Pathophysiology

Urinary tract calculi can be found in the kidney, collecting system/ureters, or bladder, and are usually composed of **calcium** (70–85% of cases). Other stones are composed of **magnesium-ammonium-phosphate** (15–20%, **struvite** or "infection" stones), *uric acid* (5–10%) or *cystine* (< 3%). Their etiology is often idiopathic, but the risk is increased in the setting of **dehydration, urinary stasis, infection, hypercalcemia,** and other **metabolic abnormalities** (e.g., hyperuricemia, cystinuria, salt imbalance due to malabsorption). Staghorn calculi *usually occur in women* due to a much greater incidence of urinary tract infections and are caused by **urease**-producing bacteria, classically *Proteus mirabilis* (*Escherichia coli* does *not* produce urease).

Diagnosis & Treatment

Stones can be asymptomatic, especially when confined to the kidney. Classic renal stone pain ("renal colic") is **abrupt in onset, severe,** and **intermittent;** located anywhere from the **flank** down to the **groin** (depends on where a stone is); and associated with **nausea and vomiting.** Patients are usually *uncomfortable no matter what position they are in* and move around frequently trying to get comfortable (unlike patients with peritonitis, who usually choose to lie as still as possible).

Physical exam is often unimpressive, though associated signs may be present with coexisting infection (e.g., costovertebral angle tenderness with upper tract infection). Hematuria on urinalysis (or a history of gross hematuria) is highly suggestive, and crystals are often seen in the urine. A *low urine pH (< 5.5) suggests uric acid stones;* a *pH of 8 suggests infection.*

Diagnosis is confirmed with an **intravenous pyelogram** or **noncontrast CT scan** (use **ultrasound** in pregnant women and kids, due to radiation concerns). Most stones (**85%**) can be seen on a plain abdominal x-ray (uric acid stones are the classic cause of radiolucent stones). Treatment is **aggressive hydration,** which allows the majority of stones to pass *spontaneously,* and **pain control,** with narcotics if needed for severe pain. Larger stones that don't pass usually need surgical intervention (i.e., endoscopy or open surgery) or **extracorporeal shock-wave lithotripsy.** Staghorn calculi generally need early, aggressive surgical management to prevent sepsis and renal function loss from obstruction.

More High-Yield Facts

Collect urine to determine stone composition. Cystine stones are *diagnostic* of **cystinuria/aminoaciduria.** Uric acid stones can usually be treated with urine **alkalinization** (e.g., sodium bicarbonate) and **reduced dietary purine.**

Urology

History

A 28-year-old man presents with a chief complaint of a "lump" in his testicle and vague abdominal pain. He says he first noticed the lump a week ago after being hit in the groin while playing basketball. The patient is concerned because the lump has not gone away, but mainly came in to see you due to nagging, vague abdominal pain and "fullness," which he says has affected his appetite. He takes no medications and has no history of dysuria, sexually transmitted diseases, vomiting, or gastroesophageal reflux–type symptoms. Past medical and family histories are noncontributory.

Exam

T: 98.9°F   BP: 118/76   RR: 14/min.   P: 68/min.

The patient is thin and athletic appearing. Head, neck, and chest exams are normal. Bowel sounds are normal. A posterior mid-abdominal mass is palpable, but without tenderness. Rectal and extremity exams are unremarkable. Genital exam reveals a palpable, nontender, solid mass in the left testicle that does not transilluminate. No urethral discharge, scrotal skin changes, or inguinal adenopathy is appreciable.

Tests

Hemoglobin: 15 g/dL (normal 14–18)
WBCs: 8000/μL (normal 4500–11,000)
Platelets: 310,000/μL (normal 150,000–400,000)
Creatinine: 0.8 mg/dL (normal 0.6–1.5)
BUN: 11 mg/dL (normal 8–25)
Urinalysis: normal
Abdominal CT scan: extensive retroperitoneal adenopathy (see figure)

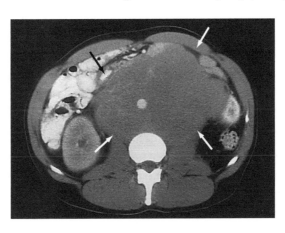

Testicular cancer with metastases to retroperitoneal lymph nodes

The CT image, at the level of the lower kidneys, demonstrates extensive, bulky retroperitoneal adenopathy (*arrows*) surrounding the aorta.

Pathophysiology

Testicular cancer is the *most common solid malignancy in males 15 to 40 years old.* Risk factors include **cryptorchidism, white race, and age.** Most cancers arise from **germ cells,** such as **seminoma** (most common); *stromal cell tumors* (e.g., Sertoli or Leydig cell tumors) are much less common. Metastatic disease to the testicle, often **lymphoma or leukemia,** is more common in **older adults.** Testicular lymphatic and venous drainage are to the **periaortic region;** thus retroperitoneal metastases is common. *Hematogenous* metastases (usually to the lung) can also occur.

Diagnosis & Treatment

Patients usually present with a **palpable, painless testicular mass,** though a history of *recent trauma* and/or *testicular pain* are not uncommon. **Symptoms of metastatic disease** (e.g., vague abdominal fullness/pain or shortness of breath) may be present at the time of diagnosis (**one-third** of cases).

Exam classically reveals a **solid, nontender, palpable testicular mass,** though tenderness may be present. Inguinal adenopathy and scrotal skin erythema or edema are *usually absent* (if present, consider infection).

Ultrasound can be used to define the mass. *Intratesticular masses are usually malignant; extratesticular masses are usually benign.* Diagnostic confirmation for malignancy is pathologic via **surgical exploration and orchiectomy** (also part of the treatment). Chest x-ray and abdominal CT are used to rule out metastases. *Yolk sac tumors* make **alpha-fetoprotein,** and *choriocarcinoma* produces **human chorionic gonadotropin** (β-HCG), both of which can be used for monitoring. The rare **Leydig-cell tumor** may cause *precocious puberty* or *feminization* (secretion of testosterone or estrogen). With metastases, seminomas are often treated with **radiation** (usually highly effective, +/− chemotherapy); "nonseminomatous" lesions are typically treated with **chemotherapy** alone.

More High-Yield Facts

Other scrotal masses: **Hydroceles** are simple fluid collections between the two layers of the **tunica vaginalis** of the testis. They may be congenital due to a **patent processus vaginalis,** or acquired (e.g., inflammation, impaired lymphatic drainage). On exam, they are *cystic-feeling,* surround the testicle, and **readily transilluminate.** No treatment is usually needed. **Varicocele** refers to enlarged veins (the **pampiniform plexus**) in the scrotum (80% of cases are on the left) that feel like a **"bag of worms."** The veins *become prominent upon standing and go away when the patient is supine.* They may cause **pain** or **infertility,** which are indications for surgical treatment.

Urology

History

A 73-year-old man seeks medical advice for low back pain and left hip pain that began several weeks ago. He also describes unintentional weight loss of roughly 15 pounds over the past few months, which he attributes to a decreased appetite. The patient mentions that he has had difficulty urinating, with occasional blood in his urine over the last few weeks. Past medical history is remarkable for hypertension and osteoarthritis. He takes terazosin, irbesartan, and rofecoxib. Family and social history are noncontributory.

Exam

T: 98.8°F   BP: 138/86   RR: 14/min.   P: 74/min.

The man is thin and and in no acute distress. Head, neck, chest, and abdominal exams are unremarkable. Genital exam is normal. Rectal exam reveals no occult blood in the stool, but the prostate demonstrates stony, hard induration, and two firm nodules are palpable. The straight leg raise maneuver does not reproduce the patient's back or hip pain, and he has a full range of back, hip, and leg motion, with no tenderness on palpation of these areas. No adenopathy is appreciated, and the neurologic and dermatologic exams are normal.

Tests

Hemoglobin: 15 g/dL (normal 14–18)
WBCs: 7700/μL (normal 4500–11,000)
Platelets: 320,000/μL
   (normal 150,000–400,000)
Creatinine: 0.8 mg/dL (normal 0.6–1.5)
BUN: 11 mg/dL (normal 8–25)
Urinalysis: 4+ hematuria;
   otherwise normal
Prostate specific antigen (PSA):
   23 ng/dL (normal < 5)
Bone scan: see figure

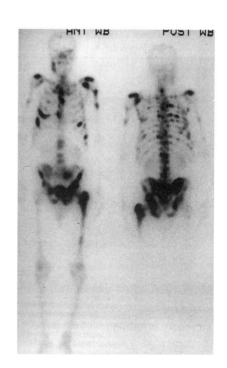

Metastatic prostate cancer

The bone scan reveals widespread metastatic disease (*dark black areas*), including involvement of the spine, ribs, pelvis, left sacral area, and the left hip and femur.

Pathophysiology

Prostate cancer is generally **adenocarcinoma** (90–95% of cases) and usually occurs in the *periphery* of the gland, making **digital rectal exam** useful in detection. Risk factors include **age, black race** (blacks > whites > Asians), and **family history.** Prostate cancer is *very rare* in those less than 40, and the incidence rises steadily after this age (**80%** of clinically diagnosed prostate cancer is in men **over age 65**). The cancer is slow-growing, making screening with PSA *controversial*. Rectal exam, however, is not controversial, since it needs to be done anyway for colorectal cancer screening. Local extension and bone metastases are the usual routes of prostate cancer spread.

Diagnosis & Treatment

Early prostate cancer is **asymptomatic** and is increasingly being detected by screening. Local symptoms occur later and include **hematuria** and nonspecific benign prostatic hypertrophy (BPH)–like symptoms, such as **urinary urgency, nocturia,** and **weakness of the urinary stream** ("nonspecific" because BPH often coexists in this patient population). A classic late presentation is **bone pain** (classically lower back) due to bony metastases.

Physical exam, if positive, classically reveals a **stony, hard prostate** and/or one or more **firm nodules** in the prostate. A markedly **elevated PSA** (> 15–20) essentially clinches the diagnosis. Mildly elevated PSA is a common clinical problem and is *a nonspecific finding that can be caused by BPH or infection.* Serum prostatic **acid phosphatase** (no longer widely used) becomes elevated only if the cancer has broken through the prostatic capsule. **Transrectal ultrasound-guided biopsy** of the prostate is often used to confirm the diagnosis and provide histologic grading (Gleason score), which is prognostically useful. **Bone scans** are ordered in the setting of *bone pain or a markedly elevated PSA* to look for metastases.

Treatment is highly variable for local disease and may include **observation** alone (85–95% 10-year survival rate; older patients often "die with, rather than from" prostate cancer), **surgery** (prostatectomy), or **radiation.** For metastatic disease, **hormonal therapy** is preferred, such as *orchiectomy, GnRH analogs* (e.g., leuprolide), or *antiandrogens* (e.g., flutamide).

More High-Yield Facts

If asked on Step 2 about screening with PSA, *discuss the risks, benefits, and limitations* of the test with a patient over age 50 (40 in blacks), and let the patient decide if he wants to be screened annually.

Urology

History

A 4-year-old boy is brought to your office by his mother for abdominal pain that began a few days ago and has gotten worse. The mother states that her son also has been somewhat lethargic, with a decreased appetite over the last few weeks, but she says he has not sustained trauma or had fever, headache, vomiting, or other symptoms. The patient was previously healthy and has no significant past medical history. He takes no medications, and his mother claims that his growth and development have been normal. Family history is noncontributory.

Exam

T: 99.1°F   BP: 124/88 (elevated)   RR: 18/min.   P: 94/min.

The patient is healthy appearing and in no acute distress. Height and weight are appropriate for age. Mild scleral pallor without scleral icterus is noted. Neck and chest exams are unremarkable. Abdominal exam reveals a large, palpable, smooth, and solid mass in the left flank and abdomen. Normal bowel sounds are heard, and the child is not tender during palpation. Rectal and genitourinary exams are negative. No musculoskleletal, neurologic, or dermatologic abnormalities are appreciated.

Tests

Hemoglobin: 10 g/dL (normal 11–13)
WBCs: 8700/μL (normal 6000–16,000)
Platelets: 330,000/μL (normal 150,000–400,000)
Creatinine: 0.7 mg/dL (normal 0.4–0.7)
BUN: 11 mg/dL (normal 5–17)
AST: 32 U/L (normal 20–60)
Amylase: 21 U/L (normal 8–79)
Calcium: 9 mg/dL (normal 8.7–9.8)
Urinalysis: 3+ hematuria; otherwise normal
Abdominal ultrasound: 9-cm intrarenal solid mass with distortion of the renal pelvis

Pathophysiology

Wilms' tumor is an embryonal renal malignancy generally seen in **children age 6 months to 7 years** (90% of cases), with a peak incidence in those *2 to 4 years old*. A **genetic defect** has been associated in some cases (familial cases and those associated with aniridia), and 5% of affected children have associated *congenital anomalies* (classically **aniridia, hemihypertrophy,** and/or **genitourinary anomalies** such as hypospadias and cryptorchidism).

Diagnosis & Treatment

Most children present with a **palpable abdominal mass** (often large) that may be noticed by the parent or discovered during a physical exam. In up to 30% of patients, varying symptoms include **abdominal pain, anemia, hematuria, anorexia,** fever, and/or malaise. Urinalysis may reveal **hematuria** (30–50% of cases), and **hypertension** and/or anemia may be present.

Diagnosis is suggested by physical exam, which usually leads to imaging with **ultrasound, CT scan, or intravenous pyelogram.** The diagnosis is confirmed with **biopsy,** and CT scan of the abdomen and chest is used to define the extent of the tumor and rule out metastases. Treatment includes **surgery** in most cases, often with **chemotherapy.** Roughly **85%** of patients are ultimately **cured.**

More High-Yield Facts

The primary differential diagnosis for Wilms' tumor is an **adrenal neuroblastoma.** Approximately **50%** of neuroblastomas arise in the adrenal medulla, with the remaining cases usually found along the **sympathetic ganglia** in the abdomen or thorax. Neuroblastoma tends to present in a younger age group (*80% occur in those < 4 years old,* and neuroblastoma accounts for 50% of malignancies seen in infancy). When arising from the adrenal gland, neuroblastoma *rarely invades the kidney* and generally *doesn't distort the collecting system* (unlike Wilms' tumor), so imaging can often suggest one diagnosis over the other. Neuroblastoma is also more likely to metastasize widely, and often presents with **bone marrow involvement** (bone marrow biopsy is part of the staging). **Elevated catecholamine levels** also are typical. Chemotherapy is the usual treatment, along with surgery. Rarely, spontaneous regression of neuroblastoma occurs.

After *CNS tumors,* neuroblastoma and Wilms' tumor are the most common primary *solid* malignancies of childhood (but **leukemia** is the most common overall malignancy in childhood).

Urology

History

You are called to perform a newborn exam 1 hour after an uncomplicated vaginal delivery at term. No difficulties were encountered by the mother during her pregnancy, and she received regular prenatal care, including a prenatal sonogram that revealed no fetal abnormalties. The mother denies any use of tobacco, alcohol, or other drugs during pregnancy, and she has no medical problems. Family history is noncontributory. APGAR scores were 9 and 9 at 1 and 5 minutes, respectively.

Exam

Vital signs: normal

The baby is active and healthy appearing. His length and weight are at the 50th percentile for age. Head, neck, chest, and abdominal exams are normal. No neurologic abnormalities are identified, and his skin appears normal. Rectal exam is unremarkable. Genital exam reveals an opening on the underside of the distal penile shaft just proximal to the glans (see figure). During the exam, the child expels urine through this opening. No other abnormalities are identified.

Tests

Hemoglobin: 18 g/dL (normal 17–22)
Creatinine: 0.7 mg/dL (normal 0.6–1.0)
BUN: 8 mg/dL (normal 5–17)
Bilirubin, total: 1.9 mg/dL (normal < 5.8)

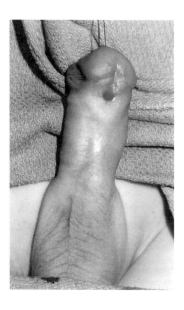

Pathophysiology

In boys with hypospadias, the urethral meatus is located abnormally on the **underside (ventral aspect) of the penis.** The urethral opening can occur anywhere along the penile shaft, or even in the scrotum or perineum in more severe cases. In girls with hypospadias (much less common than in boys), the urethra generally opens into the **vaginal introitus.** The cause of hypospadias is failure or delay in the midline fusion of the **urethral folds.**

Diagnosis & Treatment

Hypospadias is generally discovered during the newborn exam of a boy. Most cases are mild and *not* associated with additional genitourinary anomalies. With more severe degrees of hypospadias (i.e., more proximal urethral opening), there is an increased risk of associated anomalies. In most cases of male hypospadias (including mild cases), a **chordee** is present. A chordee is a ventral band of fibrous tissue that causes a *ventral* (i.e., downward) *curvature of the penis,* which is especially noticeable during an erection and may make sexual intercourse difficult or impossible later in life if not surgically corrected. Incomplete development of the **foreskin** is also common (the **"dorsal hood" deformity**).

Treatment is **surgical** correction, usually done in early childhood. The foreskin is generally used in the reconstructive surgery, so *children with hypospadias should not be circumcised.*

More High-Yield Facts

Epispadias is less common than hypospadias, and describes a urethral opening on the *dorsal* (top) aspect of the penis (again, more common in males, but can occur in females). It is associated with **exstrophy of the bladder,** which is a gap in the abdominal wall and anterior wall of the bladder that leaves the interior of the bladder exposed. Treatment is **surgical,** but the condition represents a more serious defect, and patients often have incontinence even after treatment.

Posterior urethral valves describe abnormal **congenital folds or membranes** that narrow or obstruct the *prostatic* urethra. They are almost always seen in males and are a potential cause of urinary tract obstruction and recurrent urinary tract infections (UTIs). The diagnosis is classically made with a **voiding cysto-urethrogram** performed after a *UTI* and/or *hydronephrosis* is discovered in a male child, though the condition can be detected during prenatal ultrasound in more severe cases. Treatment is **surgical** (ablation of the valves, usually done endoscopically).

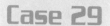

Case 29

Urology

History

A 13-year-old boy presents with a chief complaint of severe left scrotal pain, accompanied by nausea and vomiting, that began 2 hours ago. He says the pain started shortly after lifting weights at the gym, was fairly rapid in onset, is constant, and rates a 10 out of 10 in severity. The pain preceded the nausea and vomiting. The patient denies any history of fever, upper respiratory tract infection, dysuria, urinary urgency, urethral discharge, or other genitourinary symptoms. He has never experienced symptoms like this before and denies any history of scrotal or abdominal trauma. Past medical history is insignificant; vaccinations are up-to-date; and the patient takes no medications. He has never been sexually active and does not drink alcohol or use illicit drugs. The patient's father claims that he is a good student and a well-adjusted child who participates in many extracurricular activities.

Exam

T: 99°F   BP: 118/76   RR: 16/min.   P: 84/min.

The patient is athletic appearing, intelligent, oriented, and in obvious discomfort. Height and weight are appropriate for age. Head, neck, chest, and abdominal exams are unremarkable; bowel sounds are normal, and there is no abdominal tenderness. No costovertebral angle tenderness is noted. Genital exam reveals Tanner stage III sexual maturity of the genitalia and a diffusely swollen and tender left testicle. The left testicle is somewhat elevated within the scrotum compared to the right, and mild scrotal edema without significant erythema is evident. The tenderness does not improve with elevation of the left testis. You note that the right testicle has a somewhat horizontal lie within the scrotum, with the long axis oriented in the anteroposterior direction. The cremasteric reflex is absent on the left and present on the right. No inguinal hernia is detectable. The remainder of the exam is unremarkable.

Tests

Hemoglobin: 15 g/dL (normal 12–16)
Leukocyte count: 8100/μL (normal 4500–13,000)
Platelets: 270,000/μL (normal 150,000–400,000)
Creatinine: 0.9 mg/dL (normal 0.6–1.2)
BUN: 10 mg/dL (normal 8–20)
Urinalysis: normal

Pathophysiology

Torsion occurs from twisting of the spermatic cord, which can compromise testicular blood supply. Torsion is often related to the "**bell clapper deformity,**" a normal, usually bilateral, anatomic variant. Normally, tunica vaginalis covers all of the testicle except a posterior "bare area," where the testis is anchored to the posterior scrotal wall. In the bell clapper deformity, the tunica vaginalis entirely encases the testicle so that it hangs freely like a bell clapper (the inner part that strikes the side of the bell). Torsion is most often seen in *adolescents* (peak incidence in those **12–18 years old**).

Diagnosis & Treatment

Patients classically present in adolescence with **acute, sudden onset of scrotal/ testicular pain** that may be spontaneous or after exertion. **Scrotal skin swelling** then often occurs. **Nausea and/or vomiting** are also typical.

On exam the testicle is **swollen** (due to edema and reactive hydrocele formation) and **tender,** and often **rides high in the scrotum** compared to the unaffected side. Scrotal wall edema may also be seen. The tenderness is not relieved by elevation of the testis, as it classically is in epididymitis (**Prehn's sign**), though this is *not* a reliable sign. The unaffected testicle typically has a **horizontal lie** rather than the usual vertical orientation. This is an indication of the bell clapper deformity. The cremasteric reflex (stroke the inner thigh and the testicle on that side elevates) is usually *absent* on the affected side, though this sign is also not reliable (this reflex can be absent as a normal variant).

Acute, sudden onset of scrotal pain in an adolescent is torsion *"until proven otherwise"* **and is a surgical emergency.** With a typical history/exam, proceed to immediate surgical consultation/exploration to allow testicular salvage. Ultrasound is used to confirm the diagnosis before surgery only if rapidly available. If surgically treated *within 4–6 hours of symptom onset,* there is a high likelihood of testicular salvage, which drops quickly after this time period. **Bilateral orchiopexy** (to prevent future torsion on either side) and unilateral detorsion (untwisting of the spermatic cord), or orchiectomy if the testicle is not viable, are performed.

More High-Yield Facts

A history of dysuria, urethral discharge, or significant fever is generally *absent* with torsion, and should make you think of **epididymitis.** The cause is often a *sexually transmitted disease bug* (e.g., *Neisseria gonorrhoeae*) in those who are *younger/sexually active,* and a *urinary tract infection bug* (e.g., *Escherichia coli*) in *older adults.* Diagnosis can be confirmed with **urinalysis** and/or **ultrasound.** Treatment is empiric **antibiotics** to cover appropriate bugs. Epididymitis is much more common than torsion after adolescence.

Urology

History

A 63-year-old man is concerned because he has observed blood in his urine for the past 3 weeks. He has also noticed urinary frequency and urgency over the last 2 weeks, but denies pain or dysuria. Prior to the onset of these problems, the patient had no genitourinary symptoms. He denies fever, weight loss, and any history of previous urinary tract stones or infections, but admits to unusual fatigue recently. Past medical history is remarkable for hypertension, for which the patient takes hydrochlorothiazide. He has a 50-pack-year smoking history and drinks alcohol only on rare, social occasions. Family history is remarkable for hypertension and coronary artery disease.

Exam

T: 98.8°F   BP: 138/86   RR: 16/min.   P: 90/min.

The patient is thin and in no acute distress. Head and neck exam is remarkable for mild scleral pallor. Chest exam reveals scattered crackles throughout the lung, which largely clear with coughing and a slightly prolonged expiratory phase. No signs of consolidation are evident. Abdominal and rectal exams are normal, and the stool is negative for occult blood. No costovertebral angle tenderness is appreciated. The genital exam is unremarkable, as is the remainder of the exam.

Tests

Hemoglobin: 11 g/dL (normal 14–18)
Mean corpuscular volume: 78 μm/cell (normal 80–100)
Leukocytes: 7600/μL (normal 4500–11,000)
Platelets: 350,000 (normal 150,000–400,000)
Creatinine: 1 mg/dL (normal 0.6–1.5)
BUN: 11 mg/dL (normal 8–20)
Urinalysis: gross hematuria and 1+ WBCs; otherwise normal
Intravenous pyelogram and bladder ultrasound: see figures

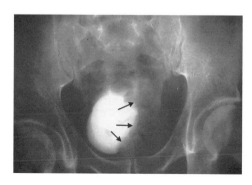
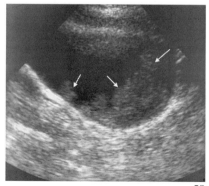

The intravenous pyelogram and ultrasound images show an irregular filling defect/mass (*arrows*) on the left side of the bladder.

Pathophysiology

Roughly 90% of bladder cancers in the U.S. are **transitional cell carcinomas** (TCC); squamous cell cancer is less common. **Age** (peak incidence at **60–70 years**), **sex** (**male:**female ratio roughly 3:1), **cigarette smoking** (causes roughly 50% of bladder cancer), **race** (**whites** affected twice as often as blacks; uncommon in Asians), and **chronic bladder irritation** (e.g., recurrent stones or infections) are the primary risk factors. Occupational exposure to *aniline dyes/aromatic amines* (e.g., rubber, chemical, textile industries), *bladder schistosomiasis* (*Schistosoma haematobium,* a cause of squamous cell carcinoma in other countries) and long-term use of *cyclophosphamide* or *phenacetin* are other risk factors.

Diagnosis & Treatment

The classic presentation is **painless hematuria,** whether gross or microscopic. **Urinary frequency, urgency,** and/or **dysuria** are also common, and suggest more diffuse or invasive disease. Nonspecific systemic symptoms (e.g., weight loss or fatigue from anemia) are less common.

Physical exam is often *normal.* Signs of anemia may be present. **Urinalysis** reveals hematuria (signs of infection usually absent; may see some urinary leukocytes from inflammation). Urine **cytology** may reveal malignant-appearing cells, and the urine may contain elevated levels of certain proteins associated with bladder malignancy (e.g., nuclear matrix protein 22). With gross hematuria or microscopic hematuria of unknown etiology that persists on short-interval follow-up, **further evaluation is needed in all patients,** *especially adults over 40 years old.* Evaluation is usually performed with **intravenous pyelogram** or **ultrasound,** with complementary **cystoscopy** (and biopsy of any suspicious areas) in *all adult patients over 50* and those with bladder cancer risk factors.

TCC spreads by local invasion, and treatment is related to the *depth of tumor invasion* (i.e., superficial vs. invasive disease) and histologic grade. Superficial tumors are generally treated with **cystoscopic ablation** or **intravesical immunotherapy/chemotherapy** (e.g., bacille Calmette-Guérin, interferon-alpha, mitomycin C) and repeated follow-up cystoscopy and urine analysis to check for recurrence. Invasive disease is treated using surgery (usually radical cystectomy) +/− chemotherapy.

More High-Yield Facts

The risk of developing a second TCC is high (5–50%); therefore, those diagnosed with TCC need routine, regular follow-up *indefinitely* (usually with annual cystoscopy and urine evaluation).

Case 31

Urology

History

A 63-year-old man has been experiencing gradual onset of difficulty urinating over the last year or so. He describes frequent problems initiating and maintaining a normal stream of urine—he feels as though he has to strain to maintain the stream—and he has a sensation of incomplete bladder emptying. In addition, the patient feels as though he has to urinate more frequently during the day, often with associated urgency. He gets up two or three times per night to urinate; 2–3 years ago this would rarely happen. He denies pain during urination, urethral discharge, fever, and weight loss. Past medical history is notable for gout, hypertension, and coronary artery disease. The patient takes allopurinol, colchicine, metoprolol, and daily aspirin. Family history is noncontributory. The patient is married and does not smoke or drink alcohol.

Exam

T: 98.5°F   BP: 140/88   RR: 14/min.   P: 66/min.

The patient is overweight, but appears comfortable. Head, neck, chest, and abdominal exams are normal. A mildly distended bladder is palpable. No neurologic, musculoskeletal, or dermatologic abnormalities are detected. No costovertebral angle tenderness is appreciated. Genital exam is unremarkable, with no urethral discharge or other abnormalities noted. Rectal exam reveals brown stool that is negative for occult blood, and an enlarged, smooth prostate gland with a rubbery consistency and loss of the normal median furrow. No prostate nodules, irregularity, or tenderness is appreciated.

Tests

Hemoglobin: 16 g/dL (normal 14–18)
Leukocytes: 7900/μL (normal 4500–11,000)
Platelets: 240,000/μL (normal 150,000–400,000)
Creatinine: 1 mg/dL (normal 0.6–1.5)
BUN: 11 mg/dL (normal 8–20)
Prostate-specific antigen (PSA): 3.6 ng/mL (normal 0–4.0)
Urinalysis: normal

Benign prostatic hypertrophy (benign prostatic hyperplasia; BPH)

Pathophysiology

Hypertrophy/hyperplasia of the **transitional zone** of the prostate (surrounds the prostatic urethra) is a normal part of aging, with histologic evidence of BPH in **90% of 80-year-old men.** If BPH is significant, it can cause symptoms due to bladder outlet/urinary obstruction. Symptomatic BPH is not seen in men under age 30, and the incidence increases steadily with age, affecting roughly **30% of men over the age of 50.** BPH does *not* predispose to the development of prostate cancer.

Diagnosis & Treatment

Symptoms of BPH can be classified as obstructive, irritative, and other. *Obstructive symptoms* include difficulty initiating the urinary stream (**hesitancy**), difficulty maintaining the urinary stream (**intermittency**), a **weak urinary stream, straining** to urinate, **terminal dribbling** of urine, and a **sensation of incomplete bladder emptying.** *Irritative symptoms* include **urgency, frequency, nocturia, incontinence,** and occasionally, dysuria. *Other symptoms* relate to **recurrent urinary tract infections, hematuria, bladder calculi, urinary retention,** and **renal failure.**

Exam may reveal a distended bladder. Rectal exam may be normal (since hypertrophy is periurethral, not peripheral), but classically reveals a **nontender, smoothly enlarged prostate** with a **rubbery consistency** and **loss of the normal median furrow.** PSA can be *normal or mildly elevated* due to increased prostatic tissue.

BPH treatment relates to symptom severity, patient preferences, and complications. With *mild symptoms,* **observation** is often appropriate. With *moderate symptoms,* medical therapy with **finasteride** (an alpha-reductase inhibitor; shrinks the gland) or **alpha-blocking agents** (e.g., terazosin, tamsulosin; relax smooth muscle in bladder neck and prostatic urethra) is beneficial. With *medical failure or complications,* **surgery** is usually advised (e.g., transurethral resection of the prostate [TURP], prostatectomy). Surgery can cause **impotence** and usually makes patients **infertile** after the procedure due to **retrograde ejaculation** (sperm goes backwards into bladder).

More High-Yield Facts

Patients with severe BPH may develop **acute urinary retention,** a urologic emergency (because it can cause renal failure). Patients have **anuria** (> 12–24 hours), suprapubic pain, urgency, and a **distended bladder** on exam; **bilateral hydronephrosis** is seen on imaging. Initial treatment is to *drain the bladder.* If a transurethral (e.g., Foley) catheter can't be passed, place a *suprapubic* catheter. After patient stabilization, surgery (e.g., TURP) is usually advised to prevent recurrence and renal function deterioration.

Case 32

Vascular Surgery

History

A 68-year-old man presents to the emergency department with a chief complaint of complete loss of vision in his left eye that began 30 minutes ago, but resolved in the last 5 minutes while he was waiting to see you. He says the vision loss occurred suddenly while he was watching television, was painless, and felt like "someone pulled a shade down over my eye." He admits to a similar episode, for which he did not seek medical treatment, a week ago. In that episode, the vision returned within 1 minute. The patient denies any other visual symptoms and has no known visual disorders. He also denies headache, scalp pain, jaw pain, and muscle pain or stiffness. There is no history of depression or past psychiatric disturbance. Past medical history is significant for hypertension and diabetes. Medications include lisinopril, atenolol, metformin, and pioglitazone. The patient has smoked roughly 1 pack of cigarettes per day for the last 40 years and drinks alcohol regularly. His family history is significant for heart attacks and strokes on his father's side.

Exam

T: 98.6°F   BP: 156/90   RR: 16/min.   P: 76/min.

The patient is alert, oriented, and pleasant. Ophthalmologic exam reveals moderate changes of diabetes and hypertension in the retina, but no macular edema, hemorrhage, or neovascularization. The pupils are equally round and reactive, and the extraocular movements are intact. Visual acuity is 20/25 bilaterally. Examination of the remainder of the cranial nerves is unremarkable. No scalp tenderness is present. Neck exam reveals a left carotid bruit. Chest exam reveals clear lungs and a normal cardiac rate and rhythm without murmurs. Abdominal and rectal exams are normal. No focal neurologic deficits are appreciated, and the extremity exam is remarkable only for slightly diminished peripheral pulses in the lower extremities.

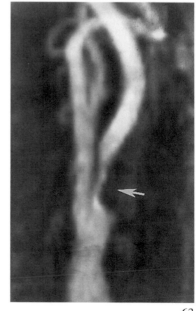

Tests

Hemoglobin: 17 g/dL (normal 14–18)
Leukocyte count: 7400/μL
  (normal 4500–11,000)
Platelets: 290,000/μL
  (normal 150,000–400,000)
Creatinine: 1.1 mg/dL (normal 0.6–1.5)
BUN: 10 mg/dL (normal 8–20)
ESR: 7 mm/hr (normal 0–20)
Magnetic resonance angiography (MRA)
  of the left carotid artery: see figure

Transient ischemic attack (TIA) with amaurosis fugax from carotid artery stenosis

The MRA reveals atherosclerotic narrowing (*arrow*) of the internal carotid artery origin (carotid bulb).

Pathophysiology

Carotid artery stenosis is usually due to **atherosclerosis** and results from the same primary risk factors as coronary artery disease: age, hypertension, diabetes, cigarette smoking, hypercholesterolemia, and family history. As the lumen of the internal carotid artery (ICA) becomes progressively irregular and narrowed, symptoms and signs of ischemia can result. Atherosclerotic plaque tends to be most bulky in the **carotid bulb,** the region that is "cleaned out" during a carotid endarterectomy (CEA).

TIA is considered to be a precursor to stroke. Only time and/or imaging can distinguish between stroke and TIA, as TIA produces the *same symptoms as a stroke* but they resolve within 24 hours (**often within 30–60 minutes**).

Diagnosis & Treatment

Patients may be *asymptomatic* or present with symptoms of a TIA or stroke. The large majority will have one or more atherosclerosis risk factors.

Physical exam classically reveals a **carotid bruit** on the affected side. Other signs may be related to generalized vascular disease (e.g., hypertensive retinopathy, diminished peripheral pulses) or TIA/stroke. In the setting of suspected carotid stenosis, **ultrasound** or **magnetic resonance angiography** is used as a screening exam. If this test shows severe stenosis, and surgical treatment is being considered, **conventional carotid angiography** is often performed because it is the *gold standard* for determining the presence and degree of carotid stenosis (the clinical trial data that showed the benefit of CEA are based on conventional angiography). If ultrasound/MRA is normal or reveals only mild disease, CEA-correctable disease is highly unlikely to be present (treat medically).

Management of carotid stenosis depends on the degree of stenosis. Patients with *less than 70%* stenosis (diameter reduction) are treated medically with **antiplatelet agents** (e.g., aspirin, clopidogrel, ticlopidine). Those with *70–99%* stenosis, with or without symptoms, benefit from **CEA** and should be offered **surgery** if they are appropriate candidates (e.g., not too many comorbidities, no previous large stroke). Note that CEA should *not* be performed on those with complete ICA occlusion. Management of those with *50–69%* stenosis and symptoms is controversial, but on Step 2 treat these patients medically.

More High-Yield Facts

Other less common causes of carotid artery narrowing include **vasculitis** (e.g., Takayasu's or temporal arteritis) and **carotid dissection,** which is usually due to trauma.

Case 33
Vascular Surgery

History

A 69-year-old woman is troubled by intermittent, severe periumbilical abdominal pain of 2-month duration. She says the pain comes on 15–30 minutes after eating, is severe and continuous, and lasts for 60–90 minutes. The patient has not been eating well because she is afraid of the pain. She thinks she has lost 15 pounds over the last 2 months because of her eating habits. The woman has tried several over-the-counter remedies for her pain, including bismuth, ranitidine, and calcium carbonate, without any pain relief. She denies jaundice, fever, melena, hematochezia, and any previous history of dyspepsia, ulcers, reflux, or abdominal pain.

Past medical history is significant for hypertension, hypercholesterolemia, coronary artery disease (CAD), previous myocardial infarction, and peripheral vascular disease. Past surgical history is significant for coronary artery bypass grafting and right lower extremity arterial bypass for severe claudication. Medications include hydrochlorothiazide, amlodipine, and atorvastatin. Social history is significant for a 50-pack-year smoking history. Family history is significant for atherosclerotic vascular disease.

Exam

T: 98.7°F   BP: 162/88   RR: 14/min.   P: 76/min.

The woman is quite thin, but pleasant, oriented, and in no acute distress. Head and neck exam reveals bilateral carotid bruits. No jaundice or scleral pallor is appreciated. Chest exam demonstrates essentially clear lungs and a normal cardiac rate and rhythm, with no cardiac murmurs or other abnormalities. Abdominal exam reveals normal bowel sounds, with no organomegaly, masses, or tenderness. Rectal and pelvic exams are normal. Stool is negative for occult blood. Extremity exam shows signs of peripheral vascular disease in the lower extremities. The remainder of the examination is unremarkable.

Tests

Hemoglobin: 15 g/dL (normal 12–16)
Leukocyte count: 6400/μL (normal 4500–11,000)
Platelets: 270,000/μL (normal 150,000–400,000)
Creatinine: 1.2 mg/dL (normal 0.6–1.5)
BUN: 13 mg/dL (normal 8–20)
AST: 10 U/L (normal 7–27)
Amylase: 60 U/L (normal 53–123)
Bilirubin, total: 0.3 mg/dL (normal 0.1–1)
ESR: 7 mm/hr (normal 0–20)
Upper GI series and barium enema: normal
CT scan of the abdomen and pelvis: normal

Mesenteric ischemia, chronic (intestinal angina)

Pathophysiology

Intestinal angina is *equivalent to cardiac angina* and is caused by **atherosclerosis.** Because of collateral blood flow between the celiac axis and superior and inferior mesenteric arteries, high-grade narrowing or occlusion of *at least two* of these arteries is usually needed to produce chronic ischemic-type symptoms. After eating, intestinal (mesenteric) blood flow increases; therefore, *having a meal is the equivalent of exercising* with cardiac angina, and results in symptoms.

Diagnosis & Treatment

Patients have **multiple atherosclerosis risk factors** and usually a history of clinically significant atherosclerotic disease in other areas (e.g., CAD, peripheral vascular disease). The classic history is **postprandial abdominal pain** that begins **15–60 minutes after eating, lasts for 1 or more hours,** and is **periumbilical and severe. Weight loss,** often severe, is due to a fear of eating (which causes pain).

Physical exam often reveals evidence of vascuar disease in other areas, but is usually *unremarkable.* Abdominal pain and tenderness are usually *absent* at presentation. The exam, lab values, and imaging studies help rule out other causes of weight loss and abdominal pain, such as **abdominal malignancy** (especially **pancreatic** or **gastric cancer**), **pancreatitis,** and **peptic ulcer disease.** The diagnosis is established with **conventional angiography of the mesenteric arteries,** which generally reveals stenosis or occlusion of at least two of the main intestinal arteries.

The preferred treatment is **surgical revascularization** (bypass), **endarterectomy** of affected vessels, or **angioplasty** (in poor surgical candidates), so blood can get beyond the areas of stenosis or occlusion to perfuse the bowel. Intervention is preferred because those left untreated are at high risk for **intestinal infarction,** which carries a high mortality rate.

More High-Yield Facts

Acute mesenteric/intestinal ischemia or infarction presents with **severe abdominal pain out of proportion to physical exam, nausea/vomiting,** diarrhea, **blood in the stool** (gross or microscopic), **leukocytosis,** and, often, an **elevated lactate level.** The cause may be *atrial fibrillation* (emboli), *thrombosis,* or a *hypotensive episode.* Vasculitis (e.g., polyarteritis nodosa) is another potential cause. Treatment is usually surgical (resection of affected bowel and/or attempted embolectomy), with or without preoperative angiography. Abdominal x-rays may reveal thickened mucosal folds (called "thumbprinting" when in the colon). Mortality is high.

Case 34

Vascular Surgery

History

A 49-year-old man presents to your office with the chief complaint of a "sore" on his left ankle. He says he first started noticing chronic skin changes around his left ankle, including scaly skin and dark discoloration, a few years ago. Roughly 2 weeks ago, he noticed that the skin was starting to break down. He also complains of chronic swelling and pain, which he describes as "heaviness," in his left leg that becomes more pronounced after prolonged standing. These symptoms often get better if he sits down and elevates his leg. The patient's chronic symptoms began roughly 2 years ago, after he sustained a left femur fracture in an automobile accident and developed a left lower extremity "blood clot," for which he received warfarin for 6 months. The patient denies fever and does not experience pain when at rest (sitting or lying down).

Past medical history is otherwise unremarkable, and the patient takes no medications other than as-needed NSAIDs for leg pain. He does not smoke or drink alcohol. Family history is noncontributory.

Exam

T: 98.8°F   BP: 124/78   RR: 14/min.   P: 78/min.

The patient is alert and oriented, and appears comfortable. Head, neck, chest, abdomen, and rectal exams are unremarkable. Peripheral pulses are normal. No sensory or motor deficits are appreciated. The left ankle is not significantly tender, and no pus or foul-smelling odor can be appreciated (see figure). Range of motion is full. You note a few mildy prominent varicose veins in the left lower extremity. When the patient is sitting with the leg dependent, mild cyanosis of the foot and ankle develop, which resolve when the leg is briefly elevated above the level of the heart. The remainder of the examination is unremarkable.

Tests

Hemoglobin: 15 g/dL
(normal 14–18)
Leukocytes: 6600/μL
(normal 4500–11,000)
Platelets: 230,000/μL
(normal 150,000–400,000)
Creatinine: 1 mg/dL
(normal 0.6–1.5)
BUN: 9 mg/dL
(normal 8–20)
ESR: 6 mm/hr
(normal 0–20)

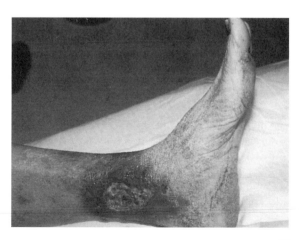

Venous stasis ulcer from chronic venous insufficiency

Pathophysiology

Chronic venous insufficiency usually occurs in the lower extremities and results from **venous valvular incompetence** in the deep venous system, with resultant *venous hypertension*. Prolonged venous hypertension leads to symptoms and skin changes. Risk factors include **deep venous thrombosis (DVT), varicose veins, trauma, and family history.**

Diagnosis & Treatment

Patients often have a history of prior DVT or varicose veins. Classic symptoms include **chronic leg heaviness or soreness made worse by long periods of standing or leg dependency,** with or without accompanying **swelling** and/or **cyanosis.** *Symptoms generally improve when the patient sits, lies down, and/or elevates the leg.*

On exam, chronic skin changes are evident, including **dark-brown skin pigmentation around the ankle** (due to hemosiderin deposition from breakdown of extravasated RBCs caused by venous hypertension), **skin induration, edema,** and a **leathery texture.** The skin is prone to become dry, scaly, and pruritic (known as **stasis dermatitis**). *Cyanosis of the extremity with dependency* (caused by venous engorgement) *that goes away with elevation* (improves venous return) *is classic.* Venous insufficiency ulcers usually occur around the **medial malleolus** of the ankle (sometimes around the lateral malleolus). The ulcerations are usually **shallow and irregular,** and contain granulation tissue. They are usually *not* painful or tender, or only mildly so, unless infection coexists (cellulitis).

The diagnosis is generally **clinical,** but **ultrasound** or **plethysmography** can be confirm venous incompetence. Perform culture of the base of the ulcer if coexisting infection is suspected, and treat with antibiotics. Treatment for the ulcer (and venous insufficiency in general) is *conservative,* with **elastic compression stockings** and **leg elevation.** Skin grafting may be needed in severe cases.

More High-Yield Facts

• *Arterial* insufficiency ulcers are due to *ischemia.* They are **very painful, focal/"punched-out" appearing,** and occur on the **underside of the foot** (below the metatarsal heads or heel) or on the **toes.** Elevation of the leg *worsens* pain (decreased blood flow). A history of claudication and/or multiple atherosclerotic risk factors is typical. Treatment is **surgical revascularization.**

• **Diabetic foot ulcers** look similar to and occur in the same location as arterial insufficiency ulcers, but are **painless** due to **neuropathy.** They result from *pressure phenomena* (not ischemia). Diabetics with foot ulcers need evaluation for arterial insufficiency though, as it may coexist.

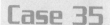

Case 35

Vascular Surgery

History

A 58-year-old man is troubled by impotence. He also complains of nagging heaviness, weakness, and pain in his buttocks, hips, and thighs whenever he tries to walk more than a few hundred feet. The pain comes on "like clockwork," but goes away when he stops to rest for a few minutes. His symptoms began roughly 2 months ago and have gotten slightly worse since then. The patient decided to come see you when he realized his impotence was not a temporary phenomenon. He denies depression and says his sexual desire is normal, but he cannot achieve erection through any means of stimulation, including masturbation. He denies chest pain, shortness of breath, fever, or other symptoms.

Past medical history is significant for hypertension and hypercholesterolemia. The patient is not taking any medications for these conditions because he usually "feels fine." He has smoked two packs of cigarettes a day for "as long as I can remember," but drinks alcohol only on social occasions. There is a strong family history of coronary artery and peripheral vascular disease, but he has never been diagnosed with either.

Exam

T: 98.5°F   BP: 168/94   RR: 14/min.   P: 82/min.

The patient is slightly overweight, but in no acute distress. Head, neck, and chest exams are unremarkable. Abdominal exam reveals normal bowel sounds and a faint bruit in the midline just below the level of the umbilicus. No tenderness is noted with palpation, and no pulsatile mass is appreciated. The femoral, popliteal, and pedal pulses are not palpable on either side. In addition, you note atrophy of the buttock muscles bilaterally. The patient is not tender to palpation of the buttocks, hips, or thighs. His lower extremities are cool, and you note shiny, atrophic-appearing skin and loss of hair below the mid-thigh bilaterally. No neurologic deficits are present, and the straight leg raise test is negative bilaterally. Genital examination is unremarkable. No rashes or other abnormalities are appreciated.

Tests

Hemoglobin: 17 g/dL (normal 14–18)
WBCs: 7000/μL (normal 4500–11,000)
Platelets: 250,000/μL (normal 150,000–400,000)
ESR: 9 mm/hr (normal 0–20)

Leriche syndrome

Pathophysiology

Leriche syndrome describes the clinical symptoms that occur with *chronic* **athero-sclerotic aortoiliac occlusion** in **men.** The occlusion generally starts near the aortic bifurcation and extends into the common iliac arteries. The symptoms are not as dramatic as you might expect because the occlusion occurs gradually in Leriche syndrome and *collateral circulation* develops. The syndrome classically describes a triad of **impotence, buttock/hip/thigh claudication,** and **atrophy of the buttock muscles.** Impotence is due to decreased blood flow to the penis secondary to reduction in *internal iliac artery* blood flow bilaterally.

Diagnosis & Treatment

Patients complain of impotence and claudication that affects the buttocks and/or the hips or thighs *bilaterally.* The impotence is physical, not psychological—patients cannot achieve an erection under any circumstance.

Examination may reveal a **bruit over the distal aorta** (in the midline at or just below the umbilicus) and may also reveal a bruit over the *common femoral arteries.* Atrophy of the buttock muscles and possibly other muscles of the lower extremities is classic. Evidence of arterial insufficiency of the lower extremities includes **shiny and atrophic/thinned skin, loss of hair,** and **cool temperature.** Femoral, popliteal, and pedal pulses are *absent bilaterally.* **Dependent erythema/ rubor** of the lower extremities with **pallor on elevation** and/or skin ulcerations/ gangrene can be seen in more severe cases when inadequate collateral circulation has developed.

The diagnosis can be solidified with **ultrasound** examination of the lower extremity arteries and is confirmed with **conventional contrast angiography.** Treatment is surgical in most patients with significant symptoms, typically via revascularization and placement of an **aortoiliac bypass graft.** Control of modifiable atherosclerotic risk factors (e.g., hypertension, cholesterol, diabetes) is an important adjunctive treatment.

More High-Yield Facts

Acute aortic occlusion is usually due to a **cardiac embolus** (watch for atrial fibrillation or a ventricular aneurysm), though it can occur from *spontaneous thrombosis,* usually secondary to complications of atherosclerosis. It is a *medical emergency* that threatens the viability of the lower extremities. **Severe pain, coolness, pallor, and pulselessness of both lower extremities** is seen. **Emergent angiography** is performed to confirm the diagnosis. Treatment is **emergency thrombectomy or revascularization.**

Case 36

Vascular Surgery

History

A 62-year-old man comes to the emergency department with severe abdominal and low back pain that began last night and has been constant. He describes the pain as deep and boring, rating it 9 out of 10 in severity. The patient denies nausea, vomiting, fever, diarrhea, jaundice, previous similar episodes of pain, melena, and hematochezia. His past medical history is significant for hypertension and hypercholesterolemia. Medications include fosinopril, nifedipine, carvedilol, and simvastatin. The patient has an 80-pack year smoking history. Family history is notable for atherosclerotic vascular disease.

Exam

T: 98.9°F   BP: 158/92   RR: 16/min.   P: 90/min.

The patient is of normal build and in moderate distress from pain. Head, neck, and chest exams are normal, except for a mildly increased expiratory phase of respiration. Abdominal exam reveals normal bowel sounds and no organomegaly. You note very prominent vascular pulsations on both sides of the midline at the level of the umbilicus. When you palpate this area to determine the extent of the pulsations, the patient complains of increased pain. No peritoneal signs are present. There is no focal tenderness to palpation of the lower back. Peripheral pulses are palpable and symmetric, though mildly decreased in the lower extremities. Rectal exam demonstrates mild, smooth prostatic enlargement, but otherwise is normal, as are neurologic and dermatologic exams.

Tests

Hemoglobin: 17 g/dL (normal 14–18)
WBCs: 7800/μL (normal 4500–11,000)
Platelets: 290,000/μL (normal 150,000–400,000)
ESR: 9 mm/hr (normal 0–20)
Abdominal CT scan: see figure
Abdominal x-ray: see figure

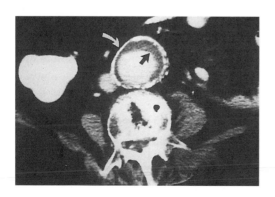

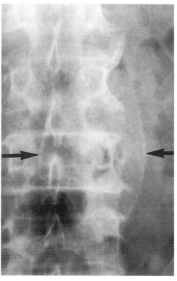

Abdominal aortic aneurysm (AAA)

The x-ray shows curvilinear mural calcifications (*arrows*) in an AAA. On CT, the AAA has mural calcifications (*white arrow*) and intraluminal thrombus (*black arrow*).

Pathophysiology

Aortic aneurysms can involve any part of the aorta, but about *75%* involve the abdominal aorta (i.e., AAA), and *90%* of these begin below the level of the take-off of the renal arteries. Aneurysms may end before the aortic bifurcation or extend into one or both iliac arteries. Risk factors for AAA include **male gender, age, smoking, hypertension,** and **family history.** Less commonly, AAA can be due to **infection** (usually due to *Staphylococcus aureus, Salmonella,* or fungal infection), **arteritis,** or **trauma.** The feared complication of AAA is spontaneous rupture (which carries a very high mortality even in the setting of immediate treatment), the risk of which *increases with an increasing AAA diameter.*

Diagnosis & Treatment

Patients are most often *asymptomatic.* Vague **low back pain** or perception of pulsations in the abdomen is occasionally present. With rapid AAA expansion or impending rupture, patients may have **severe low back or abdominal pain,** often described as **constant, deep,** and **boring** in nature.

Exam reveals a prominent **pulsatile abdominal mass** (i.e., prominent aortic pulsations), usually around *the level of the umbilicus in the midline,* which may be very difficult to feel in obese individuals. The aneurysm may be **tender** due to rapid expansion, aneurysm leakage, and/or impending rupture. In the setting of rupture, **hypotension and/or shock** is generally present.

If hypotension or shock is present, a pulsatile abdominal mass should prompt immediate laparotomy in an attempt to prevent death. In a stable patient who is symptomatic, a **CT scan of the abdomen and pelvis with IV contrast is** performed to confirm the diagnosis and evaluate the characteristics of the AAA. **Ultrasound** is a cheaper, but still accurate alternative to measure aneurysm size in asymptomatic patients or monitor a known AAA. Plain x-rays may reveal curvilinear wall calcifications. In asymptomatic persons, elective AAA repair is advised for all who can tolerate surgery if the maximal AAA diameter is ≥ **6 cm** (due to a *50% risk of rupture in the next year*) and for healthier persons if the AAA is ≥ **4–5 cm** (25% risk of rupture in the next year). An AAA ≤ **4–5 cm** is followed with periodic imaging (e.g., every 6 months) to monitor for enlargement.

More High-Yield Facts

Popliteal aneurysms (70% are bilateral) have a high association with AAA, and if detected should prompt imaging to screen for an AAA.

Case 37

Vascular Surgery

History

A 24-year-old man has suffered a crush injury of his left leg, which resulted in a comminuted, closed tibial fracture and multiple skin abrasions. He has no other identifiable injuries. Though the patient admits to significant pain, he is fairly stoic and refuses all pain medicine besides acetaminophen. His past medical history is insignificant, and he takes no regular medications. In the emergency department, the patient's skin is thoroughly cleansed, and after stabilization, reduction, and casting, he is admitted to the hospital.

Several hours later, you are called to see the patient for increasing leg pain.

Exam

T: 99°F   BP: 128/82   RR: 18/min.   P: 92/min.

The patient is alert and oriented, but crying out in pain when you enter the room. He says his pain is now "11 out of 10" and complains of alternating tingling and numbness in his left leg and foot. You examine the cast and see that the skin around the edges of the cast is swollen. The patient's exposed toes demonstrate mild cyanosis. You split the cast open down to the skin and pry it open to allow examination of the leg, which results in resolution of the toe cyanosis. The leg feels firm and swollen, much more so than upon admission, and the overlying skin is shiny and smooth. Pedal pulses in the left foot are palpable and fairly symmetric compared to the right foot. Sensation and two-point discrimination are decreased in the left foot compared to the right—these findings were not present on admission. Passive flexion and extension of the foot results in excruciating pain, which the patient describes as "10 times worse than when I got to the hospital," and he refuses to actively flex or extend the foot.

Tests

Hemoglobin: 16 g/dL (normal 14–18)
WBCs: 7800/μL (normal 4500–11,000)
Platelets: 320,000/μL (normal 150,000–400,000)
Ultrasound of left lower extremity: negative for deep venous thrombosis

Pathophysiology

Muscle compartments are enclosed by fascia and can develop **increased internal pressure** that may result in compartment syndrome. The cause is usually an increase in the contents of the compartment from **hemorrhage or edema,** such as occurs after **trauma** (usually a *tibial or supracondylar humeral fracture, electrical burn, crush injury,* or *surgery*) or **ischemia** (arterial occlusion or reperfusion injury after restoration of blood flow, classically *after a surgical revascularization procedure*). Alternatively (or additionally), **restriction** of a muscle compartment can be causative (e.g., application of *compressive dressing or tight cast*). In either mechanism, the increased pressure in the compartment can impair venous return and cause ischemia and more fluid leakage into the compartment, further increasing intracompartmental pressure and resulting in a vicious cycle. Complications include *muscle necrosis* and *permanent nerve damage* (e.g., Volkmann's contracture).

Diagnosis & Treatment

Patients should have the appropriate traumatic, surgical, or ischemic history. Symptoms typically occur in the **leg or forearm,** though other areas can be involved. Symptoms include **pain on passive movement that is out of proportion to the injury** and **paresthesias** (i.e., tingling and/or numbness).

On exam, the affected muscle compartment usually **feels firm and/or tensely swollen** and the **overlying skin is shiny and smooth. Decreased sensation and two-point discrimination** occur at a slightly later stage and are due to the pressure effects on sensory nerves in the affected compartments. *Pulses are usually normal* or only slightly decreased, but if they are markedly decreased or absent, this is a late, ominous sign requiring immediate intervention. **Cyanosis** and/or **delayed capillary refill** may be present at this stage. **Paralysis** is another late sign that may be irreversible.

If other symptoms are present in the right clinical setting, the development of decreased pulses or neurologic symptoms should prompt **immediate fasciotomy** (incising the muscle compartment to relieve the pressure and prevent/reduce permanent damage to muscles and nerves). In less urgent cases (no neurologic symptoms), **measure intracompartmental pressures** (e.g., with a needle manometer) to confirm the clinical diagnosis. With pressures **> 30 mmHg,** fasciotomy is generally indicated.

More High-Yield Facts

The four Ps of compartment syndrome: **pain, paresthesias, paralysis,** and **pulselessness.** However, paralysis and pulselessness are late findings—diagnosis and treatment should occur *before* these two signs occur.

Case 38

Vascular Surgery

History

A 63-year-old woman complains of intermittent pain and muscle fatigue, of 3-month duration, in her left calf. She describes the pain as "achy" and "crampy." The pain seems to always occur after she walks up the stairs in her two-story house and goes away if she stops to rest for a minute. If she continues to walk and doesn't rest when the pain comes on, the pain and fatigue worsen until she is forced to stop and wait for them to pass. The patient denies calf pain at rest, fever, trauma, and similar symptoms in the right leg. Her past medical history is notable for hypertension, diabetes, and hypercholesterolemia. Medications include candesartan, propranolol, metformin, insulin, and niacin. The patient has a 40-pack year smoking history and drinks alcohol regularly. She is physically inactive and admits that walking up the stairs in her house once or twice a day is probably her only exercise. Family history is noncontributory.

Exam

T: 98.4°F   BP: 158/92   RR: 14/min.   P: 72/min.

The patient is alert and oriented, thin, and in no acute distress. Head, neck, and chest exams are unremarkable, with a regular cardiac rate and rhythm noted and no murmurs appreciated. Abdominal exam is normal, as are rectal and pelvic exams. No neurologic deficits are appreciated, and sensation is intact and symmetric in the lower extremities. The left femoral pulse is diminished and the popliteal and pedal pulses are not palpable, though they can be detected with a Doppler probe. Delayed capillary refill is noted in the left toes. The right lower extremity pulses and capillary refill are normal. The skin of the left lower leg is cool, atrophic, and shiny compared to the right leg, and the skin of the left foot is dry and scaly, though normal on the right. In addition, the toenails on the left foot are thickened and brittle compared to the right.

Tests

Hemoglobin: 15 g/dL (normal 12–16)
WBCs: 6800/μL (normal 4500–11,000)
Platelets: 290,000/μL
  (normal 150,000–400,000)
Glucose: 142 mg/dL
  (normal fasting 70–110)
Angiogram of the left iliac artery:
  see figure

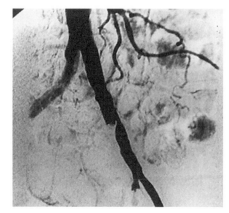

Claudication

The angiogram shows high-grade stenosis of the left common iliac artery (the triangular-shaped filling defect in the center of the image).

Pathophysiology

Claudication is the **skeletal muscle/extremity equivalent of angina** and is usually due to atherosclerosis. The risk factors for peripheral vascular disease (PVD) are the same as those for coronary artery disease, with **smoking** and **diabetes** the most potent modifiable risk factors. Upon exercise of the lower leg muscles—usually during walking—athersclerotic, stenotic arteries can't dilate to increase blood flow/oxygen delivery to the muscles, resulting in **ischemia that resolves with rest.**

Diagnosis & Treatment

Patients classically describe **pain, aching, cramping, and/or fatigue** in the **calf muscles** after walking a certain, *reproducible distance.* Claudication severity is often described clinically by the walking distance needed to cause symptoms (e.g., "four-block claudication"), allowing objective comparison to future/past claudication severity.

On exam, **pulses are decreased and/or absent** starting at a level above the affected muscles. Other signs of PVD include **thin, atrophic, cool, and shiny skin,** which is often **dry and scaly,** with **diminished or absent hair growth** and **thickened, brittle toenails.** In addition, *pallor* of the affected foot may be noted after 1 or 2 minutes of leg *elevation,* followed by *dependent rubor / erythema.* With more severe arterial insufficiency, *ulcers* may develop on the underside of the foot (usually below the metatarsal heads or on the heel) or tips of the toes. **Necrosis, gangrene,** and/or **rest pain** (*constant pain at rest,* usually in the **fore-foot,** that is *aggravated by leg elevation* and relieved by hanging the foot over the edge of the bed or sitting in a chair with the foot dependent) occur with very severe disease and indicate a **high risk of limb loss.** Ultrasound or **angiography** (the gold standard) can confirm the diagnosis.

Treatment depends on symptom severity. For mild symptoms, aggressive reduction of atherosclerosis risk factors (e.g., treat diabetes, stop smoking) and an **exercise program** are the preferred treatments. **Pentoxifylline** or **cilostazol** are second-line adjunctive therapies to reduce symptoms (via various mechanisms). With more severe symptoms/signs, **angioplasty** and/or **surgical bypass** may be needed. With rest pain, ulceration, or gangrene, surgery or angioplasty is usually needed to save the limb.

More High-Yield Facts

Prophylactic foot care is an important measure in PVD, and includes *daily foot inspection* (with prompt reporting of abnormalities), *keeping feet clean and lubricated,* and *wearing comfortable shoes that fit well.*

Neurosurgery

History

A 72-year-old woman is brought in by her daughter, who thinks her mother may have Alzheimer's disease. The daughter says the patient has become extremely and uncharacteristically forgetful over the past 3 months, and is unable to remember most things for more than a few seconds. In addition, the daughter claims that her mother has become somewhat paranoid and hostile, often accusing other family members of stealing her things. The patient has also become incontinent of urine over the last several weeks, and this is now occurring on a daily basis. Lastly, the daughter mentions that her mom started walking "funny" a few weeks ago. The daughter says that her mother was her normal, perky, intelligent, witty, and active self 3 months ago, but now seems like a totally different person. She does not think her mother is depressed and has not noticed her acting sad or crying. The patient's appetite has not changed and she seems to be sleeping well.

Past medical history is essentially unremarkable. The patient has seen a doctor only once or twice in the last 20 years. She takes no medications and does not smoke or drink alcohol. There is no family history of dementia or psychiatric illness.

Exam

T: 98.6°F   BP: 138/82   RR: 14/min.   P: 72/min.

The patient is alert and knows her name, but does not know where she is or what the date is. She is unable to remember any of three words you ask her to remember after 5 minutes have elapsed. When you ask the patient to walk to evaluate her gait, you notice that she has a very hesitant, ataxic gait and a broad-based stance when she starts and stops walking. However, she seems to walk fairly well in between her trouble starting and stopping. The remainder of the neurologic exam reveals only bilateral extensor plantar responses (bilaterally positive Babinski signs). No cogwheel rigidity, hyperreflexia, or muscle atrophy is noted. The patient is incontinent of urine during the exam. The rest of the exam is unremarkable.

Tests

Hemoglobin: 14 g/dL (normal 12–16)
WBCs: 6600/μL (normal 4500–11,000)
Sodium: 140 meq/L (normal 135–145)
Potassium: 4 meq/L (normal 3.5–5)
Calcium: 9.5 mg/dL (normal 8.5–10.5)
Creatinine: 0.9 mg/dL
Glucose: 82 mg/dL (normal fasting 70–110)
CT scan of the brain: abnormally enlarged ventricles with minimal age-related atrophy; otherwise normal
Lumbar puncture: normal

Pathophysiology

NPH is a poorly understood disorder that is related to a ***communicating* hydrocephalus,** which is thought to be due to *poor cerebrospinal fluid (CSF) reabsorption by the arachnoid villi and/or subarachnoid space obliteration.* Roughly 50% of patients relate a history of meningitis, subarachnoid hemorrhage, and/or head trauma, but in the remainder no such history is obtainable. NPH is a disorder of the **elderly** and is generally *not seen in those less than 50 years old.*

Diagnosis & Treatment

The classic triad of NPH is an ataxic gait, urinary incontinence, and dementia. These symptoms generally come on *gradually* over weeks or months and can mimic Alzheimer's dementia. The rapidity in onset (weeks or months versus years) and fairly characteristic gait abnormality, however, argue against Alzheimer's. A history of head trauma, infection, or hemorrhage is often obtainable.

The gait is classically described as **hesitant,** with patients having *trouble stopping and starting movement,* and **ataxic.** A **broad-based stance** is often present. Common dementia-type symptoms include **short-term memory loss, lack of orientation,** and **personality changes / psychiatric disturbances.** Bilateral extensor plantar responses (i.e., **positive Babinski signs**) are classically described, though not always present. CT scan or MRI of the brain reveals **abnormal ventricular enlargement,** and a lumbar puncture is typically *normal* (no increased pressure or evidence of infection). Other confirmatory tests are variable in their reliability (e.g., nuclear cisternography) and are unlikely to be asked about on Step 2.

The primary treatment is **surgical shunt placement** to drain off CSF, usually a *ventriculoperitoneal* shunt, which causes symptom improvement in about 50% of patients. NPH is one of the few *potentially reversible* causes of dementia.

More High-Yield Facts

Obstructive **hydrocephalus** has multiple causes and often presents fairly dramatically, with acute or subacute onset of severe headache, lethargy, and sometimes coma. Focal neurologic deficits and/or signs of increased intracranial pressure (e.g., **papilledema**) are often present. Perform CT scan or MRI of the brain to look for a tumor or other abnormality. Lumbar puncture (avoid with signs of increased intracranial pressure or obvious tumor on CT scan or MRI) usually reveals an abnormally **elevated opening pressure.** Treatment is directed at the underlying cause.

Neurosurgery

History

A 51-year-old woman is brought to the emergency department by emergency medical services for a seizure witnessed by her husband. The patient is currently post-ictal, so the husband provides the history. He says his wife was sitting on the couch watching television with him when she suddenly started convulsing on the floor, with twitching in all her extremities. She did not respond to his voice or attempts to "wake her up." She also was incontinent of urine during the episode. The patient has no history of similar episodes or seizures.

The husband feels guilty for not bringing his wife in to see a doctor weeks ago, as she had been complaining of severe headaches and numbness and tingling sensations in her right leg for a few weeks. The patient apparently did not want to see a doctor, however. He also states that his wife has been acting odd lately, often overly aggressive or inappropriate in social settings. Past medical history is unremarkable, with no history of seizures, psychiatric disorders, malignancy, hypertension, infection, or fever. The patient takes no medications and does not smoke, drink alcohol, or use illicit drugs.

Exam

T: 98.6°F   BP: 158/88   RR: 14/min.   P: 62/min.

The patient is disoriented and somnolent, but rousable with verbal stimuli. Eye exam reveals blurring of the disc margins bilaterally. The pupillary exam is normal, and the patient does not mind when you shine your penlight into her eyes. The cranial nerve examination is limited due to the patient's reduced ability to cooperate, but is normal. Her neck is supple, and her chest is clear to auscultation, with a normal cardiac rate and rhythm and no murmurs evident. Abdominal and dermatologic exams are normal. The patient seems to have grossly decreased sensation and mild hyperreflexia in the right lower extremity compared to the left.

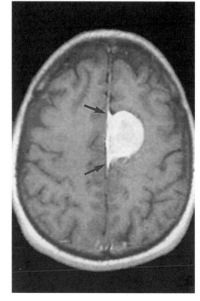

Tests

Hemoglobin: 14 g/dL (normal 12–16)
WBCs: 8600/μL (normal 4500–11,000)
MRI of the brain with contrast: fairly large, left parasagittal tumor that appears to be broadly attached to and arising from the dura mater (see figure)

Meningioma

The MRI reveals a homogeneously enhancing mass in the left parasagittal area that is attached by a broad base to the dura mater (*arrows*).

Pathophysiology

Meningiomas are generally **benign** neoplasms that arise from meningeal cells (of the arachnoid); thus they usually occur directly adjacent to the brain or spinal cord. Meningiomas occur more commonly in **women** and in those **over age 40** (classically those aged 40 to 60, but older adults and children can also be affected). Though the tumors are usually benign (there are several histologic sub-types, some of which are more aggressive), their location can result in cata-strophic consequences in some patients.

Diagnosis & Treatment

Symptoms vary depending on the location and growth pattern of the tumor. The symptoms/signs will not help you distinguish between meningioma and other pri-mary or metastatic brain tumors. Symptoms of **increased intracranial pressure** include **headache** and **vomiting** (classically projectile). Varied mental symptoms (e.g., drowsiness, personality or behavioral changes, psychotic episodes) and other neurologic symptoms may also occur from the increased pressure, or may be due to the location of the tumor. **New-onset seizures** are classic.

On exam, **papilledema** is the classic finding that suggests increased intracranial pressure. *If papilledema is present, do not perform a lumbar puncture, as you may precipitate uncal herniation and death.* Signs of infection are generally absent. **Focal neurologic symptoms** and **altered levels of consciousness** or **personality changes** are common. In the setting of a suspected mass lesion, a **CT scan or MRI of the brain with contrast** is ordered to confirm the diagnosis and deter-mine the location and imaging characteristics of the tumor. Imaging characteris-tics sometimes allow a specific diagnosis without biopsy; this is often the case with meningiomas. Meningiomas are intimately **associated with the dura** and classically occur in the **parasagittal region** or **over the convexities,** though many other locations are possible. They often demonstrate **dense, homogeneous con-trast enhancement** and may contain **calcifications.**

Treatment is **surgical resection** when possible, which is often curative. Menin-giomas that are not surgically accessible often respond to **radiation** to some degree.

More High-Yield Facts

In adults, most brain tumors are supratentorial (i.e., cerebral hemispheres), while in kids they are more often infratentorial (i.e., brainstem and cerebellum). **Glioblastoma multiforme** and **metastatic tumors** (e.g., **lung, breast**) are the most common adult brain tumors (roughly equal incidence).

Neurosurgery

History

A 71-year-old man with known prostate cancer that has metastasized to the spine, pelvis, and ribs is brought to the emergency department by ambulance for severe weakness and diminished sensation in the lower extremities. He also mentions that he feels as though he has lost some of his ability to control his bladder and bowels. Severe lower back pain over the last 5 weeks often awoke him at night, but he says his other symptoms did not begin until a week ago. The patient's oncologist told him the low back pain was due to a metastasis in the spine. At first the patient thought his weakness and sensation changes were related to the increasing number of morphine pills he was taking for pain, but when he stopped taking his pain medicine for 24 hours, the symptoms persisted. Other than prostate cancer, for which the patient had a radical prostatectomy and is currently being treated with leuprolide, past medical and surgical history is noncontributory. The patient is scheduled to start an experimental chemotherapy regimen next week.

Exam

T: 98.8°F   BP: 138/82   RR: 16/min.   P: 72/min.

The patient is alert and oriented, but essentially unable to stand up due to severe bilateral lower extremity weakness. Head and neck exams are normal. His chest is clear to auscultation, and his cardiac rate and rhythm are regular. Abdominal exam is unremarkable. Examination of the patient's back reveals severe focal tenderness with palpation of the thoracolumbar junction of the spine. He has diminished sensation below the mid-thigh region bilaterally, and significant, fairly diffuse muscular weakness in both lower extremities. Hyperreflexia is noted below both knees, and the Babinski sign is positive bilaterally. Rectal exam reveals poor anal sphincter tone and decreased sphincter control.

Consider your first step in the management of this patient.

Tests

Hemoglobin: 11 g/dL (normal 12–16)
WBCs: 8200/µL (normal 4500–11,000)
Platelets: 340,000/µL (normal 150,000–400,000)
Sodium: 137 meq/L (normal 135–145)
Potassium: 4.1 meq/L (normal 3.5–5)
Creatinine: 1 mg/dL (normal 0.6–1.5)

Subacute spinal cord compression secondary to metastatic disease

Pathophysiology

Tumors that compress the spinal cord include **metastatic lesions** (usually **lung, breast,** or **prostate**) to the spine that cause mass effect on the cord (i.e., extradural location) or **primary tumors** that arise adjacent to the spinal cord (e.g., meningioma, schwannoma). **Trauma,** severely **herniated or ruptured intervertebral disks,** and epidural or subdural **abscesses** and **hematomas** are other common causes of spinal cord compression. This condition must be diagnosed promptly, because *the ultimate neurologic prognosis and outcome are highly correlated with pre-treatment function.*

Diagnosis & Treatment

Acute spinal cord compression is usually from acute **trauma,** and presents with fairly rapid (minutes to hours) or immediate neurologic deficit after an injury. *Subacute cord compression* often occurs in patients with an appropriate history (e.g., malignancy, fever, back pain) over days to weeks. The initial symptom is usually **localized spinal pain** that classically **wakes patients up** in the middle of the night and may be made *worse* by lying down (both characteristics are uncommon with "benign" causes of back pain). Symptoms of nerve root compression (pain, weakness and/or sensory loss in a specific region) may follow. Eventually, **sensory loss and weakness of the extremities** and **incontinence of urine and/or feces** develop.

Severe **focal spinal tenderness** usually indicates metastatic disease or an intraspinal abscess. **Sensory loss,** reflex changes indicating an upper motor neuron lesion (**hyperreflexia, positive Babinski sign**), and **weakness** in the lower extremity muscles (upper extremities affected by a cervical cord lesion) are classic. **Poor anal sphincter tone** or **loss of sphincter control** may also be present. In this setting (and in this case), the first step is to give **high-dose intravenous corticosteroids** (e.g., dexamethasone), which have been shown to improve outcome. The second step is to confirm the diagnosis and characterize the cause/extent of the lesion, generally with **MRI.**

Treatment depends on the cause. Metastatic disease is usually treated with **radiation;** surgery is employed for radioresistant tumors. Hematoma, abscess (most commonly due to *Staphylococcus aureus*), and disk herniation/rupture generally require **surgical intervention** (plus antibiotics with an abscess).

More High-Yield Facts

Acute spinal cord injury (trauma) patients should also receive **immediate high-dose intravenous corticosteroids,** which can improve outcome.

Neurosurgery

History

A 24-year-old man presents with a chief complaint of altered sensation and weakness. He claims that he has decreased sensation in his shoulders and upper arms and associated weakness in these same muscle groups. His symptoms began several weeks ago on the left side with sensory changes, which gradually progressed to involve the opposite side, and were followed by gradual onset of motor weakness, which the patient says is worse on the left. He denies pain, fever, headache, trauma, seizures, weight loss, and night sweats. Past medical history is unremarkable. The patient takes no medications and doesn't use illicit drugs. Family history is noncontributory.

Exam

T: 98.7°F   BP: 118/74   RR: 14/min.   P: 70/min.

The patient is alert and oriented, with a normal mental status, and is not toxic appearing. Full ophthalmologic and cranial nerve exams are unremarkable. Bilateral atrophy and weakness of the shoulder girdle and upper arm muscles are noted, worse on the left, with associated diminished reflexes in these areas. In addition, you note loss of pain and temperature sensation over the back of the neck, upper back, shoulders, and upper arms. However, fine touch and vibration sense is preserved in these regions. The remainder of the neurologic exam is normal. Chest, abdominal, genital, rectal, and dermatologic exams are normal.

Tests

Hemoglobin: 15 g/dL (normal 14–18)
WBCs: 7700/μL (normal 4500–11,000)
Platelets: 260,000/μL (normal 150,000–400,000)
Creatinine: 1 mg/dL (normal 0.6–1.5)
ESR: 8 mm/hr (normal 0–20)
MRI of the spine: see sagittal image

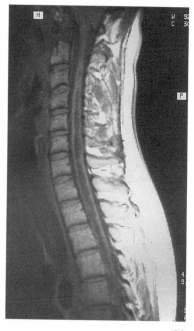

Syringomyelia

The MRI image shows an extensive cavity in the cervical and thoracic cord (the dark portion within the brighter-appearing cord).

Pathophysiology

Syringomyelia describes an **abnormal fluid-filled cavitation** of the spinal cord. It can be **idiopathic** or due to **developmental** factors (e.g., associated with the Arnold-Chiari malformation), prior **trauma,** or **tumors** affecting the spinal cord. Because the cavitation often begins in the central cervical spinal cord adjacent to the central canal, gradually increasing in size, *a fairly specific order and distribution of neurologic symptoms occurs* in the classic presentation, due to progressive involvement of different spinal cord tracts.

Diagnosis & Treatment

This is an uncommon disorder; therefore, you need only recognize the classic clinical presentation (you don't need to know how to read the MRI, and it's unlikely you'll be shown one on Step 2). Symptoms can be asymmetric, but **bilateral involvement eventually occurs** in most cases. Patients classically complain of **altered/loss of pain and/or temperature sensation** (e.g., may have a burn or injury and not feel it) in the **upper extremities** (initially upper arms and shoulders, then extending to the neck and distal arms and hands). Muscular weakness in this same distribution occurs in the next stage.

On exam, pain and temperature sensation is diminished or absent in the back of the neck, shoulders, and arms (upper arms and perhaps lower arms and hands). However, proprioception (fine touch and vibration sense) is intact in these same areas. This **classic "cape-like" distribution of unusual sensory deficits** should immediately make you think of syringomyelia. **Lower motor neuron signs** (e.g., weakness, decreased or absent reflexes, atrophy, and fasciculations) involving muscles in the same distribution may be found **in later stages** of the condition. If the cavity expands further up or down the cord, cranial nerve or thoracic involvement may occur.

The history and clinical findings in a classic case are very specific. **MRI** of the spine is used to confirm the diagnosis, characterize the extent of the syrinx, and attempt to determine the cause (e.g., neoplasm or an Arnold-Chiari malformation).

Treatment is **surgical decompression** of the cord via shunting of the cavity, akin to shunt placement used to treat hydrocephalus.

More High-Yield Facts

The most common primary intraspinal (intramedullary) tumors (which can cause syringomyelia) are **astrocytomas** and **ependymomas.**

Case 43

Cardiothoracic Surgery

History

A mother brings her 4-month-old daughter to the emergency department after the child's second episode of "turning blue" in the past week. The mother states that both episodes occurred after the infant had been crying vigorously and lasted for approximately 2–3 minutes. During both episodes, the child breathed more and more rapidly and became increasingly cyanotic until she eventually passed out. The baby was born at term after an uneventful pregnancy and had been "doing well" according to the mother, though she was told 2 months ago that the child had a murmur during a routine office visit. The child's past medical history is otherwise unremarkable.

Exam

Vital signs: normal

The child is alert, but has a cyanotic tint to her tongue and lips, which the mother says developed over the last several weeks. Weight is at the 5th percentile for age; length and head circumference are at the 25th percentile. Pupillary and neuro-logic examinations are normal. Chest exam reveals clear lungs. Cardiac rate and rhythm are normal, but there is a loud systolic ejection murmur heard along the upper left sternal border. Abdominal and neurologic exams are normal, and motor development is as expected for age. Extremity exam reveals mild clubbing of the fingernails. Pulse oximetry on room air is 88%.

Tests

Hemoglobin: 18 g/dL (normal 10–14)
WBCs: 9600/μL (normal 6000–17,500)
Creatinine: 0.3 mg/dL (normal 0.2–0.4)
Chest x-ray: mildly enlarged heart, with an upturned cardiac apex and a concavity of the left heart border at the level of the main pulmonary artery, giving the heart a "boot-shaped" appearance
EKG: sinus rhythm with right axis deviation and evidence of right ventricular hypertrophy

Pathophysiology

Tetralogy is a classic board question on all of the USMLE exams and describes a tetrad of findings: **ventricular septal defect, pulmonic stenosis** (or atresia in severe cases), an **"overriding" aorta** (i.e., receives blood from both right and left ventricles), and **right ventricular hypertrophy** (RVH). Tetralogy of Fallot (TOF) is the most commonly encountered cyanotic congenital heart defect after the neonatal period. Associated conditions include a right-sided aortic arch, patent ductus arteriosus, and Down syndrome. Clinical severity is closely correlated with the degree of right ventricular outflow obstruction.

Diagnosis & Treatment

Patients may be cyanotic and symptomatic shortly after birth or not until later in infancy, but most children present with symptoms **before the age of 2.** Parents usually become aware that the child has a problem because of **cyanosis, failure to thrive,** and/or **"tet" spells**—the classic findings in children who present in infancy or childhood. During a tet spell, which typically occurs *after vigorous crying or exertion,* the child becomes increasingly **anxious, cyanotic, and tachypneic** for a few minutes and may then develop **lightheadedness, syncope, or convulsions.** Older children classically learn to **squat down to relieve dyspnea** (because this increases peripheral vascular resistance and pulmonary blood flow).

Exam typically reveals **central cyanosis** (i.e., involves **tongue, lips, earlobes**) and a **systolic ejection murmur best heard at the upper left sternal border,** which is due to the pulmonic stenosis. **Clubbing** of the fingernails is common as well. Hemoglobin and hematocrit are often *markedly elevated,* which is a physiologic response to prolonged hypoxia (i.e., secondary polycythemia). X-ray ("boot-shaped" heart) and EKG findings (RVH) are described in the present case. **Ultrasound or MRI** confirm the diagnosis.

Treatment is **surgical correction.** Patients need **endocarditis prophylaxis** before surgical procedures for life (even after surgical correction). There is an *increased risk of sudden death* after repair (likely from arrhythmias).

More High-Yield Facts

Remember the **five Ts** of cyanotic congenital cardiac anomalies (though there are others): **TOF, transposition of the great arteries, total anomalous pulmonary venous return, truncus arteriosus,** and **tricuspid atresia.**

When pulmonary outflow obstruction is severe, the patient may *need* a patent ductus arteriosus to survive (use **prostaglandin E_1** to help keep it open).

Case 44

Cardiothoracic Surgery

History

A 62-year-old man is concerned about a change in his chronic cough—it is is now productive. He says he saw streaks of blood in his whitish sputum twice in the last 24 hours and is experiencing increased shortness of breath. The patient also mentions that his voice has become hoarse over the last few weeks, but denies fever, night sweats, chest pain, and sick contacts. Past medical history is significant for hypertension, for which he takes metoprolol. The patient has smoked two packs of cigarettes a day for the last 40 years and thinks he may have lost some weight recently.

Exam

T: 98.8°F   BP: 148/90   RR: 20/min.   P: 84/min.

The patient is mildly dyspneic, somewhat cachectic, and barrel chested. Head and neck exams are unremarkable. Chest exam reveals a prolonged expiratory phase. In addition, localized wheezing and signs of consolidation are present over the right upper lung field. Abdominal exam is unremarkable, with normal bowel sounds and no palpable organomegaly or masses. Rectal, musculoskeletal, and neurologic exams are normal.

Tests

Hemoglobin: 14 g/dL (normal 14–18)
WBCs: 8500/μL (normal 4500–11,000)
Platelets: 310,000/μL (normal 150,000–400,000)
Creatinine: 1 mg/dL (normal 0.6–1.5)
Chest x-ray: see figure

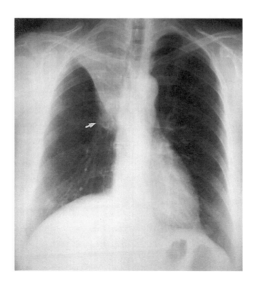

Lung cancer, likely bronchogenic carcinoma (BC)

The x-ray shows **right upper lobe collapse,** with downward bowing of the medial aspect of the minor fissure from a central mass (*arrow*)—this is the "**reverse S sign of Golden.**"

Pathophysiology

The four subtypes of BC are **squamous** (20–30%, central, may cavitate); **adeno-carcinoma** (30–40%, peripheral, most likely type in *non-smokers, bronchiolo-alveolar* subtype resembles pneumonia on x-ray); **small cell** (25%, oat cell, central); and **large cell** (15%, anaplastic cells). BC is caused by **cigarette smoke** (**90%** of cases) and rarely by asbestos, nickel, radon, coal, chromium, arsenic, uranium, or radiation exposure. BC is the *leading cause of cancer death in both men and women.*

Diagnosis & Treatment

Classic symptoms include **cough** (or *change* in smoker's cough), **localized wheezing, hemoptysis, chest pain** (chest wall invasion), and **weight loss.** Metastases may cause the presenting symptoms (e.g., bone pain, brain metastasis). A **solitary pulmonary nodule** *in those older than 40* and **pneumonia** that *fails to resolve* with treatment or *recurs in the same spot* are also suspicious.

On exam, signs of an **effusion** (malignant) or **consolidation** (atelectasis or complicating pneumonia) may be present. Blood-tinged sputum or frank hemoptysis also may be present. There are seemingly endless classic BC consequences. A central or apical (i.e., **Pancoast**) tumor can cause **Horner's syndrome, superior vena cava syndrome** (facial redness/plethora and edema from caval obstruction), **hoarseness** (recurrent laryngeal nerve involvement), and unilateral diaphragmatic paralysis (phrenic nerve). Paraneoplastic syndromes are systemic sequelae (not related to anatomy) and include **Cushing syndrome** (ACTH-secreting small cell carcinoma), syndrome of inappropriate antidiuretic hormone secretion (small cell tumors), **hypercalcemia** (squamous cell tumors) and the **Eaton-Lambert syndrome** (myasthenia gravis–like symptoms that spare the eyes).

Diagnosis is often suggested on **chest x-ray,** with **CT scan** and/or **bronchoscopy** used for further evaluation. Biopsy determines the most meaningful clinical histological distinction: **small cell,** or **non-small cell** (the other three subtypes of BC lumped together). Due to **early metastasis,** small cell cancer is treated with **chemotherapy** (classically a **platinum-based** regimen) and/or radiation. Surgical resection is often attempted in non-small cell cancers (cancer spread to major structures outside the lung, contralateral nodes, and/or distant sites precludes surgery).

More High-Yield Facts

Screening for lung cancer, even in high-risk patients, is *not* currently recommended (though CT screening trials are ongoing).

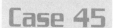

Case 45

Cardiothoracic Surgery

History

A woman brings in her 8-week-old infant with Down syndrome for a routine check-up. She mentions that the child has become somewhat short of breath over the last few weeks. He has otherwise been doing well. The mother denies fever, cough, sick contacts, jaundice, seizures, and cyanosis. The boy was delivered vaginally without complication at term, after an uneventful pregnancy. The mother denies the use of alcohol, tobacco, or other drugs during pregnancy.

Exam

Vital signs: significant for mild tachypnea and tachycardia

The child is alert and has typical facies and morphologic features of Down syndrome. Height, weight, and head circumference are all just below the 3rd percentile for age. Head and neck exams are otherwise unremarkable, as are the neurologic, abdominal, dermatologic, and rectal exams. There are no findings to suggest dehydration. Chest exam reveals clear lung fields and mild tachypnea. Cardiac rate and rhythm are regular. There is a loud, high-frequency, harsh, pansystolic murmur heard best at the lower left sternal border. No other abnormalities are detectable.

Tests

Hemoglobin: 15 g/dL (normal 9–14)
WBCs: 9600/μL (normal 6000–17,500)
Creatinine: 0.3 mg/dL (normal 0.2–0.4)
BUN: 6 mg/dL (normal 5–17)
Chest x-ray: moderate cardiomegaly, primarily of the left ventricle, with mild pulmonary venous prominence

Pathophysiology

VSD, a defect in the septum separating the two ventricles, is the most common congenital heart defect. VSD is associated with **Down syndrome** (and other trisomies), **maternal alcohol use,** other congenital anomalies, and **TORCH** infections (toxoplasmosis, other [congenital syphilis and viruses], rubella, cytomegalovirus, and herpes simplex virus). Isolated VSDs result in a left-to-right shunt.

Diagnosis & Treatment

A VSD murmur is often detected during the initial newborn examination in the nursery, when symptoms are typically absent. Symptoms may develop any time during infancy with a more severe VSD, classically at 4–8 weeks old when pulmonary resistance decreases, which increases the existing left-to-right shunt and pulmonary blood flow.

On exam, a **loud, high-pitched, harsh, holosystolic murmur heard best at the lower left sternal border** is typical. Signs of **congestive failure** (e.g., tachypnea, tachycardia, symmetric crackles in the lung bases) may be present in more severe cases. Chest x-ray may reveal **cardiomegaly** with **left ventricular enlargement** with or without x-ray signs of congestive failure. The diagnosis is confirmed with **echocardiography,** which is not always initially needed for soft or mild murmurs (that are likely to go away). MRI or diagnostic cardiac catheterization may be needed in more complex cases (i.e., other associated cardiovascular anomalies).

Roughly **15%** of VSDs are large enough to **require therapeutic intervention.** The remaining **85%** are either **too small** to have a significant hemodynamic effect or **close spontaneously** in the first 1–2 years of life. Before considering surgery with symptomatic disease, a trial of medical therapy is usually attempted (**diuretics, salt restriction**). If medical measures fail to prevent symptoms, surgical correction/closure of the VSD is often needed.

More High-Yield Facts

VSD can be part of the **VACTERL** syndrome (vertebral, anorectal, cardiovascular, tracheoesophageal, renal and/or limb anomalies), which can be due to **trisomy 18, maternal diabetes,** or **birth control pill** use.

"Innocent" murmurs (i.e., **harmless,** requiring no treatment or expensive workup) are common in younger children. They are generally **short** and **soft** (grade 1–2), and usually occur during **systole.** The **cervical venous hum** is slightly different in that it is a **continuous, soft** murmur heard best near the upper sternal borders and under the clavicles. The cause is turbulent flow in the jugular veins; thus **the murmur can be stopped by lightly pressing on the jugular.** This feature can help distinguish the cervical hum from the somewhat similar-sounding murmur of patent ductus arteriosus.

Cardiothoracic Surgery

History

A 58-year-old man presents to the emergency department with severe chest pain that began suddenly an hour ago. He says the pain is excruciating, like nothing he has ever felt before. It is centered over the region of the heart, extending through to his back; does not involve his jaw or arms; and is not associated with shortness of breath. He describes the pain as "ripping" and says that at one point several minutes ago, it seemed to move slightly lower down in his chest.

Past medical history is notable for hypertension, which the patient admits has been poorly controlled secondary to his noncompliance with treatment regimens. He is supposed to be taking metoprolol and hydrochlorothiazide, but says he ran out of these medications a few weeks ago. The patient has smoked heavily for the last 20 years. Family history is notable for hypertension and cardiovascular disease.

Exam

T: 98.5°F   BP: 192/100   RR: 18/min.   P: 88/min.

The patient is somewhat diaphoretic and in obvious discomfort from pain. Head and neck exams are unremarkable, with no jugular venous distension noted. Chest exam reveals clear lung fields and a normal cardiac rate and rhythm; no murmurs are appreciated. Chest wall and abdomen are nontender, and bowel sounds are normal. Extremity, dermatologic, musculoskeletal, and neurologic exams are normal. Rectal exam reveals stool that is negative for occult blood.

Tests

Hemoglobin: 16 g/dL (normal 14–18)
WBCs: 10,600/μL (normal 4500–11,000)
Creatinine: 1 mg/dL (normal 0.6–1.5)
BUN: 12 mg/dL (normal 8–25)
Creatine phosphokinase (CPK):
45 U/L (normal 17–148)
CPK-MB fraction: < 5%
EKG: normal sinus rhythm with borderline changes of left ventricular hypertrophy, but otherwise negative
Chest x-ray: upper normal heart size, no evidence of infiltrate or vascular congestion, slightly widened mediastinum compared to chest x-ray 1 year ago
Chest CT scan: see figure

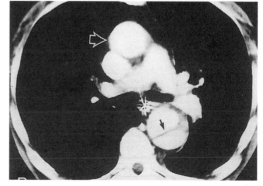

Aortic dissection

The CT scan reveals an intimal flap (*small arrow*) in the descending aorta and a normal ascending aorta (*large arrow*).

Pathophysiology

In an aortic dissection, blood enters the wall of the aorta through a tear in the intimal layer, then dissects into the media of the vessel, displacing part of the media and the intima from the remainder of the wall. The underlying abnormality is usually degenerative changes in the media, most commonly due to **hypertension,** which is associated in **70%** of cases. Other risk factors include **Marfan's syndrome** (a major cause of mortality in these patients), **coarctation of the aorta, bicuspid aortic valves,** and **iatrogenic injury.**

Diagnosis & Treatment

The classic presentation is acute onset of **severe chest pain,** which is often decribed as "**ripping**" or "**tearing**" and may **radiate to the back** (interscapular area). Diaphoresis, shortness of breath, and neurologic (from brain or spinal cord ischemia) or other symptoms related to ischemia from the dissection (bowel, renal, or cardiac ischemia) are variably present.

Patients have variable blood pressure, but most older patients have a history of hypertension. On exam, findings can be fairly normal. Signs of **heart failure and aortic regurgitation** may be present with proximal dissections involving the aortic valve. **Asymmetric pulse deficits** are classic. Neurologic and ischemic signs are variable. EKG and cardiac enzymes help exclude cardiac ischemia (a more common cause of chest pain). Chest x-ray classically shows **mediastinal widening,** but is unreliable for diagnosis (i.e., can't exclude dissection if the chest x-ray is normal).

The diagnosis is made with **CT scan** or **transthoracic/transesophageal echocardiography.** The important clinical distinction is between **proximal** (begin in ascending aorta) and **distal** (begin in descending aorta, generally distal to the left subclavian artery) dissections. Conventional angiography (the historic gold standard) is rarely used to make the diagnosis today, but may help with preoperative planning.

Proximal dissections are considered a **surgical emergency** and are treated with **immediate repair,** as 95% die within 1 year (most in first week) if treated medically (versus 25% with surgery). *Distal dissections* are treated medically with **immediate blood pressure lowering** (e.g., using nitroprusside and beta blockers), as 70% survive 1 year with medical therapy; surgical intervention is used for specific complications or done on an elective basis.

More High-Yield Facts

On Step 2, a history of **Marfan's** (or Ehlers-Danlos) syndrome **plus chest pain is dissection** until proven otherwise.

Case 47

ENT Surgery

History

A 28-year-old woman presents to the emergency department with a history of severe headache. She says the headache began 3 days ago, is fairly constant, and is in the frontal and facial areas bilaterally. She describes it as a "pressure" and also mentions occasional sharp pains in an upper tooth on the left side of her mouth. The patient also complains of nasal congestion and a yellowish-green nasal discharge that began around the time her headache started. The patient denies neurologic symptoms. Past medical history is remarkable only for a "cold" the woman had last week. The patient takes no medications and denies the use of alcohol and illicit drugs. She smokes one-half pack of cigarettes per day. Family history is noncontributory.

Exam

T: 99.6°F   BP: 116/70   RR: 14/min.   P: 68/min.

The patient is healthy appearing and in no acute distress. Examination reveals tenderness over the left cheek and adjacent to the left side of the nose. Her nasal mucosa is hyperemic and edematous. No adenopathy is appreciated in the head or neck, and the neck is supple, with no photophobia evident. The oropharynx and teeth are unremarkable, as is the remainder of the exam.

Tests

Hemoglobin: 13 g/dL (normal 12–16)
WBCs: 9600/μL (normal 4500–11,000)
Facial x-ray: see figure

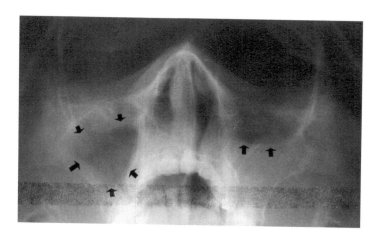

Acute sinusitis

The x-ray reveals an air-fluid level in the left maxillary sinus (*arrows*) and mucosal thickening on the right (*arrows*).

Pathophysiology

Acute sinusitis is typically a bacterial infection, though viral and fungal agents can be causative. The most common organisms are *Streptococcus pneumoniae, Haemophilus influenzae,* and *Moraxella catarrhalis.* Predisposing conditions are numerous and include upper respiratory tract infections (URI), exposure to irritants (e.g., **tobacco smoke,** air pollution), **allergy, asthma,** and impairment of mucociliary clearance (e.g., **cystic fibrosis,** anatomic abnormalities such as severe nasal septal deviation or nasal polyps).

Diagnosis & Treatment

A typical history includes a **headache,** classically frontal, which is often described as **pressure-like or throbbing.** The location partly depends on the affected sinuses, as *maxillary* sinus pain is usually in the forehead, face/cheeks, and may involve the teeth; *frontal* sinus pain is over the eyes and forehead; and *sphenoid* pain is classically a deep, retro-orbital pain. A **purulent nasal discharge** is another classic symptom that is not seen with simple viral URIs (e.g., colds) and is often accompanied by complaints of nasal congestion. Low-grade fever and **preceding URI symptoms** (e.g., sore throat, runny nose, malaise) are also common.

Exam classically reveals **tenderness over the affected sinus(es)** (in this case, over the maxillary sinus) and **erythematous and edematous nasal mucosa.** Low-grade **fever** is common. The diagnosis is generally made clinically, without the need for confirmatory imaging. Sinus/facial x-rays can visualize sinus opacification and confirm resolution. CT scans are used to evaluate patients with chronic or recurrent sinusitis and those with suspected complications (e.g., extension of infection outside the sinuses).

Treatment for *acute cases* is empiric **antibiotics** for **10–14 days** to cover typical bugs (e.g., amoxicillin/clavulanate or second-generation cephalosporin). In *chronic cases,* antibiotics are less effective, must be used for **4–6 weeks,** and should be tailored to culture results. **CT evaluation** is usually performed in chronic cases to exclude correctable anatomic abnormalities. Surgical intervention may be helpful for patients who fail repeated attempts at medical therapy.

More High-Yield Facts

Sinusitis can extend into adjacent bone (subperiosteal abscess, osteomyelitis), the orbit, and the intracranial space. Fortunately, meningitis, intracranial abscess, dural sinus thrombosis, and orbital cellulitis are rare complications. Order a CT scan if compications are suspected.

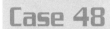

Case 48

ENT Surgery

History

A 52-year-old man is troubled by left facial numbness that began 2 days ago and is accompanied by excessive tear formation. The patient also notices that his face looks "funny" in the mirror, especially when he smiles. He had been watching televsion, when suddenly he felt a mild burning sensation behind the left ear (which is now gone), followed by facial tingling and numbness. He denies eye pain, visual disturbances, headache, fever, weight loss, other neurologic symptoms, sick contacts, and any history of similar symptoms. He claims to be a "couch potato" and has not been camping or engaged in any other outdoors activity recently. Past medical history is unremarkable, though he had just gotten over a cold when the symptoms started. The patient does not smoke, drink alcohol, or use illicit drugs, and has been sexually active only with his wife over the last 30 years.

Exam

T: 98.9°F   BP: 132/84   RR: 14/min.   P: 76/min.

The patient is mildly overweight, pleasant, and in no acute distress. On exam, you note flattening of the left nasolabial fold and a slight left facial droop. He is unable to completely close the left eye or wrinkle his left forehead. With smiling, an obvious asymmetry of the face is noted. When asked to try, the patient is unable to whistle, which he claims he can usually do. On hearing testing, he says that things sound louder in his left ear, which is not typical for him. Sense of smell and extraocular movements are intact. Pupillary and funduscopic exams are normal. No sensory loss is demonstrable. Ear, nose, and throat exams are unremarkable. No skin lesions or other neurologic deficits are identified. The remainder of the exam is normal.

Tests

Hemoglobin: 16 g/dL (normal 14–18)
WBCs: 7700/μL (normal 4500–11,000)
Platelets: 300,000/μL (normal 150,000–400,000)
Brain CT scan: normal

Pathophysiology

Bell's palsy describes **idiopathic facial nerve paralysis** and is typically **unilateral (90%** of cases). Most cases are now thought to be due to reactivation of a latent **herpes simplex I** virus infection. Nerve inflammation results in symptoms and signs of a *lower* motor neuron nerve lesion. Roughly **75%** of patients **recover** completely **without treatment,** typically within 3–12 weeks.

Diagnosis & Treatment

Patients classically complain of **facial numbness or heaviness** (though sensory loss is often not demonstrable) of fairly **rapid onset** (often a few hours to a few days). Other classic complaints are "My face looks funny," **trouble eating** (food collects between cheek and gum on affected side), and excessive tear formation. Patients actually have **epiphora** (spillage of tears onto the cheek due to drainage difficulty, which in Bell's is due to lid muscle paresis) and not excessive tear formation. Lastly, **hyperacusis** (sounds are louder on the affected side due to **stapedius muscle paralysis**) can occur. Occasionally, patients complain about the normal (uninvolved) side of their face, thinking it looks "twisted" compared to the expressionless, paralyzed side.

On exam, findings of a **7th cranial nerve paresis/paralysis** are present. Remember that the forehead muscles are *involved* with a lower motor neuron lesion such as Bell's, but typically *spared* in an upper motor neuron lesion (e.g., stroke, some brain tumors). The involved half of the face is flat and expressionless. A **facial droop, flattening of the nasiolabal fold,** and **inability to whistle, wrinkle the forehead, or completely close the eye** are typical findings on the affected side. Sensory loss often *cannot* be demonstrated on the affected side. No skin or ear vesicles are noted, which should make you think of the **Ramsay-Hunt syndrome** (herpes *zoster* reactivation, which typically also causes hearing loss and/or vertigo from 8th cranial nerve involvement).

Diagnosis is usually **clinical.** Treatment is slightly controversial, with some favoring **no treatment** and others favoring **corticosteroids** and/or antiviral herpes therapy (e.g., **acyclovir**). Use **artificial tears** (i.e., saline eye drops) to prevent **corneal damage** if an inability to close the eye is present.

More High-Yield Facts

There are many causes of facial nerve paralysis: stroke, tumor, **Lyme disease,** middle ear/mastoid infections, trauma, leukemic infiltration, multiple sclerosis, sarcoidosis, diabetes, and AIDS. Order **CT scan** or **MRI** to rule out serious causes of 7th nerve palsy with **forehead sparing, slowly progressive symptoms,** or **other neurologic findings.**

Pediatric Surgery

History

A 4-week-old infant is brought to the emergency department by his mother for persistent vomiting. He began occasionally vomiting after feeding a week ago, but has progressed to vomiting after every meal. The mother says he has a good appetite and always seems hungry, but vomits forcefully a few minutes after every attempt at feeding. She denies fever, diarrhea, and bile-stained vomitus, but thinks he is not gaining weight. The child was delivered vaginally at term without complication after an uneventful pregnancy. He is her first and only child. The mother denies the use of tobacco, alcohol, and other medications and drugs during her pregnancy. The baby is not receiving any medications and was healthy until 1 week ago.

Exam

Vital signs: tachycardia; otherwise normal

The child looks healthy and alert, but overly thin. Head exam reveals a slightly sunken anterior fontanelle. The mucous membranes are dry. No pharyngeal erythema, ear abnormalities, or lymphadenopathy is appreciated. His chest is clear to auscultation and, other than a regular tachycardia, the cardiac exam is unremarkable. On abdominal exam, you palpate a 2- to 3-centimeter, oval, firm mass, which is movable and seemingly nontender, in the right epigastrium. Rectal and genitourinary exams are unremarkable. No rash, neurologic deficits, or other abnormalities are appreciated during the remainder of the exam.

Tests

Hemoglobin: 14 g/dL (normal 11–15)
Platelets: 270,000/μL
  (normal 150,000–400,000)
Chloride: 90 meq/L (normal 95–110)
Abdominal x-ray and upper GI series:
  see figures

WBCs: 9700/μL (normal 6000–17,500)
Sodium: 135 meq/L (normal 135–145)
Potassium: 3.3 meq/L (normal 3.5–5.5)
CO_2: 34 mmol/L (normal 17–27)

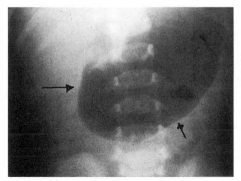
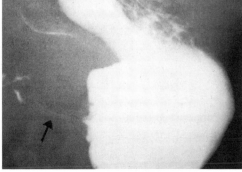

Pyloric stenosis

Plain x-ray shows marked air distention of the stomach (*arrows*) with minimal bowel gas otherwise. Barium x-ray reveals two long, thin lines of barium (*arrow*) representing contrast in the elongated pyloric canal (**"double-track" sign,** similar to the "string" sign, which is only one line).

Pathophysiology

Pyloric stenosis, also called hypertrophic pyloric stenosis (HPS), is a form of **gastric outlet obstruction** due to hypertrophy of the muscular pylorus of the stomach. It is **idiopathic,** though a family history of HPS is present in roughly 10% of cases, and typically **develops after birth. Males** are affected much more commonly than females (4:1 ratio) and term infants more often than premature infants.

Diagnosis & Treatment

Infants classically present between the ages of **2 and 6 weeks** and are almost always **asymptomatic at birth** (distinguishes HPS from congenital atresia). Patients develop **nonbilious vomiting** (classically described as forceful or **projectile**) after attempted feedings, which gets worse and becomes more frequent over time. This results in **poor or absent weight gain** and failure to thrive. Infants **do not act ill,** however, and have an **excellent appetite** and no signs of infection (e.g., no fever).

On exam, signs of **dehydration** are common. A **palpable oval** (classically described as **"olive-shaped"**), **2- to 3-centimeter, firm, movable "mass"** is usually felt in the **right epigastrium** (at least 70% of cases), representing the hypertrophied pylorus. Sometimes, peristaltic waves are visible over the epigastrium. Lab exam classically reveals a **hypochloremic metabolic alkalosis.** Plain abdominal radiographs often demostrate a distended stomach and a paucity of distal bowel gas from the obstruction.

Though *not needed in a classic case,* the diagnosis can be confirmed with **ultrasound** (preferred) or an **upper GI series.** After dehydration and electrolyte imbalance are corrected with **intravenous fluids,** surgery is generally recommended (**pyloroplasty**).

More High-Yield Facts

Gastroesophageal reflux disease is a common cause of occasional infant vomiting/"spitting up" and is partially related to physiologic immaturity of the lower esophageal sphincter (i.e., goes away with age). Vomiting is rarely forceful. Patients usually **gain weight** and are **not dehydrated.** Respiratory symptoms, including apnea, and failure to thrive can occur in some cases, however, and mandate treatment. Diagnosis is usually with an upper GI series, though an **intraesophageal pH probe** is the gold standard. Treat with smaller-size feedings, head of the crib elevation, and antireflux drugs. Surgery (fundoplication) is rarely needed.

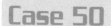
Pediatric Surgery

History

An 18-month-old boy is brought in by his father for bleeding from his rectum. The father says the bleeding occurred a few hours ago, was fairly profuse, and was mixed with blood clots. He noticed it when he changed the child's diaper. Apparently, this is the second time this has happened to the child in the last week. He says his son did not appear to be having abdominal pain during either episode and has not been ill or irritable lately. The child's appetite is good and he has been gaining weight appropriately. The father denies easy bruising, other episodes of bleeding, fever, diarrhea, vomiting, and other symptoms. The child has no significant past medical history, and his development has been progressing normally. He receives no medications and likes to eat a variety of foods. Family history is noncontributory.

Exam

Vital signs: normal

The child is active and looks healthy and alert. No scleral pallor is appreciated, and there are no signs to suggest dehydration. No bruises or skin findings are appreciated. Head, neck, and chest exams are normal. Abdominal exam is also normal, with no tenderness or masses appreciated and normal bowel sounds. Rectal exam reveals bright red blood in the rectum, but no fissure is appreciated and no tenderness is noted. A nasogastric tube is passed without difficulty for diagnostic purposes, and an aspirate is negative for blood. Neurologic and extremity examinations are unremarkable.

Tests

Hemoglobin: 11 g/dL (normal 11–13)
WBCs: 8700/μL (normal 6000–17,000)
Platelets: 290,000/μL (normal 150,000–400,000)
Stool smear: normal
Abdominal x-ray: normal
Barium enema: normal

Pathophysiology

During development, the **yolk stalk (omphalomesenteric** or **vitelline duct)** connects the gut (i.e., ileum) to the yolk sac. This connection is normally obliterated by the 7th week of gestation, but if the portion adjacent to the ileum persists, an MD is said to exist. MD is usually asymptomatic, but can cause problems related to **anatomic obstruction** (e.g., small bowel obstruction, intussusception, volvulus) or due to **heterotopic gastric tissue** (present in only 25–50% of MDs, but *responsible for nearly all cases that present with a GI bleed*), which can ulcerate and bleed.

Diagnosis & Treatment

The classic patient is **6 months to 2 years old,** though others can be affected. In these *classic young patients,* the primary complaint is **painless, profuse rectal bleeding** (often bright red blood with clots). In *older children and adults,* **symptoms of obstruction,** especially abdominal pain and vomiting, are likely to predominate, though blood in the stool is still fairly common. Signs of infectious diarrhea (e.g., fever, diarrhea, poor appetite, white blood cells and/or ova, parasites or pathologic bacteria in the stool) are absent. Barium enema, if performed, is negative, which excludes intussusception (usually causes abdominal pain and vomiting). MD causes a *lower* GI bleed, so a **nasogastric aspirate** will be **negative for blood.** No anal fissure is felt on rectal exam.

The diagnosis is difficult, but remember that there are not very many causes of GI bleeds in infants, and MD is common. Differential in this age group includes intussusception, infectious diarrhea, foreign body, arteriovenous malformation, and anal fissure. Peptic ulcer disease, gastritis, and varices are also common, but cause *upper* GI bleeds (positive blood in nasogastric aspirate). Confirmation of the diagnosis is typically done with a **nuclear medicine scan** using a radionuclide (technetium-99m pertechnetate, exam commonly called a "Meckel's scan") that accumulates in gastric mucosa, which is found in roughly 90% of MD cases that cause bleeding. Treatment is **surgical resection** of the diverticulum.

More High-Yield Facts

The **rule of twos** for MD: affects **2% of the population,** usually presents **before 2 years of age,** occurs **within 2 feet of ileocecal valve,** is **2 inches in length,** and symptoms are **2 times as common in males.**

In children < 2 years old, intussusception is usually *idiopathic.* In older children and adults, intussusception is more often caused by an anatomic "**lead point,**" which is most commonly MD in the pediatric age group.

CASE INDEX

Vascular Surgery

Neurosurgery

Cardiothoracic Surgery

ENT Surgery

Pediatric Surgery

FIGURE CREDITS

Case 1

From Klintworth GK: The eye. In Rubin E, Farber JL (eds): Pathology, 3rd ed. Philadelphia, Lippincott-Raven, 1999, pp 1537–1565; with permission.

Case 3

From Vander JF: Diabetic retinopathy. In Vander JF, Gault JA (eds): Ophthalmology Secrets, 2nd ed. Philadelphia, Hanley & Belfus, Inc., 2002, pp 341–346; with permission.

Case 5

From Gault JA: The red eye. In Vander JF, Gault JA (eds): Ophthalmology Secrets, 2nd ed. Philadelphia, Hanley & Belfus, Inc., 2002, pp 65–78; with permission.

Case 7

From Maguire JI: Age-related macular degeneration. In Vander JF, Gault JA (eds): Ophthalmology Secrets, 2nd ed. Philadelphia, Hanley & Belfus, Inc., 2002, pp 329–334; with permission.

Case 8

From Duker JS: Retinal arterial obstruction. In Vander JF, Gault JA (eds): Ophthalmology Secrets, 2nd ed. Philadelphia, Hanley & Belfus, Inc., 2002, pp 347–352; with permission.

Case 10

Left, From Klintworth GK: The eye. In Rubin E, Farber JL (eds): Pathology, 3rd ed. Philadelphia, Lippincott-Raven, 1999, pp 1537–1565; with permission.

Right, From Shield CL: Retinoblastoma. In Vander JF, Gault JA (eds): Ophthalmology Secrets, 2nd ed. Philadelphia, Hanley & Belfus, Inc., 2002, pp 365–369; with permission.

Case 14

From Collins AJ: Musculoskeletal imaging. In Provenzale JM, Nelson RC (eds): Duke Radiology Case Review. Philadelphia, Lippincott, 1998, pp 229–287; with permission.

Case 16

From Helms CA: Skeletal trauma. In Brant WE, Helms CA (eds): Fundamentals of Diagnostic Radiology. Philadelphia, Lippincott Williams & Wilkins, 1999, pp 997–1023; with permission.

Case 17

From Math KR, Cushner FD: Extremity trauma. In Katz DS, Math KR, Groskin SA (eds): Radiology Secrets. Philadelphia, Hanley & Belfus, Inc., 1998, pp 435–452; with permission.

Case 19

From Levin TL, Math KR: Pediatric skeletal radiology. In Katz DS, Math KR, Groskin SA (eds): Radiology Secrets. Philadelphia, Hanley & Belfus, Inc., 1998, pp 403–411; with permission.

Case 20

From Math KR, Ghelman B: Musculoskeletal infection. In Katz DS, Math KR, Groskin SA (eds): Radiology Secrets. Philadelphia, Hanley & Belfus, Inc., 1998, pp 293–300; with permission.

Case 21
From Inbody SB: Radiculopathy and degenerative spine disease. In Rolak LA (ed): Neurology Secrets, 3rd ed. Philadelphia, Hanley & Belfus, Inc., 2001, pp 99–110; with permission.

Case 22
From Katz DS, Perlmutter S: Urinary tract tumors. In Katz DS, Math KR, Groskin SA (eds): Radiology Secrets. Philadelphia, Hanley & Belfus, Inc., 1998, pp 190–198; with permission.

Case 24
From Resnick MI, Schaeffer AJ: Urology Pearls. Philadelphia, Hanley & Belfus, Inc., 2000, pp 66–67; with permission.

Case 26
From Daffner RH: Overview and principles of diagnostic imaging. In Clinical Radiology: The Essentials, 2nd ed. Baltimiore, Williams & Wilkins, 1999, pp 1–39; with permission.

Case 28
From Kay R: Hypospadias. In Resnick MI, Novick AC (eds): Urology Secrets, 2nd ed. Philadelphia, Hanley & Belfus, Inc., 1999, pp 177–179; with permission.

Case 30
Both figures from Katz DS, Perlmutter S: Urinary tract tumors. In Katz DS, Math KR, Groskin SA (eds): Radiology Secrets. Philadelphia, Hanley & Belfus, Inc., 1998, pp 190–198; with permission.

Case 32
From Nahum E, Murphy KD: Carotid imaging. In Katz DS, Math KR, Groskin SA (eds): Radiology Secrets. Philadelphia, Hanley & Belfus, Inc., 1998, pp 487–494; with permission.

Case 34
From McCarthy III WJ, et al: The veins and venous disease. In James EC, Corry RJ, Perry Jr JF (eds): Principles of Basic Surgical Practice. Philadelphia, Hanley & Belfus, Inc., 1987, pp 453–466; with permission.

Case 36
Left, From Williams JE, Marshall MW: Vascular radiology. In Brant WE, Helms CA (eds): Fundamentals of Diagnostic Radiology. Philadelphia, Lippincott Williams & Wilkins, 1999, pp 571–613; with permission.

Right, From Brant WE: Abdomen and pelvis. In Brant WE, Helms CA (eds): Fundamentals of Diagnostic Radiology. Philadelphia, Lippincott Williams & Wilkins, 1999, pp 651–667; with permission.

Case 38
From Murphy KD: Thrombolytic therapy. In Katz DS, Math KR, Groskin SA (eds): Radiology Secrets. Philadelphia, Hanley & Belfus, Inc., 1998, pp 510–517; with permission.

Case 40
From Liu DPC: Brain neoplasms: Primary and metastatic. In Katz DS, Math KR, Groskin SA (eds): Radiology Secrets. Philadelphia, Hanley & Belfus, Inc., 1998, pp 349–358; with permission.

Case 42

From Armstrong RM: Myelopathies. In Rolak LA (ed): Neurology Secrets. Philadelphia, Hanley & Belfus, Inc., 2001, pp 111–119; with permission.

Case 44

From Eber CD: Lung cancer. In Katz DS, Math KR, Groskin SA (eds): Radiology Secrets. Philadelphia, Hanley & Belfus, Inc., 1998, pp 77–83; with permission.

Case 46

From Williams JE, Marshall MW: Vascular radiology. In Brant WE, Helms CA (eds): Fundamentals of Diagnostic Radiology. Philadelphia, Lippincott Williams & Wilkins, 1999, pp 571–613; with permission.

Case 47

From Zeifer B: Sinusitis. In Katz DS, Math KR, Groskin SA (eds): Radiology Secrets. Philadelphia, Hanley & Belfus, Inc., 1998, pp 535–542; with permission.

Case 49

From Frush DP: Pediatric radiology. In Provenzale JM, Nelson RC (eds): Duke Radiology Case Review. Philadelphia, Lippincott-Raven, 1998, pp 411–467;with permission.

Notes

Notes

Notes

Notes

Notes

Notes

Notes

Notes

Notes

Notes

Notes

Notes

Notes

Notes

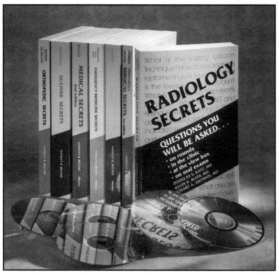

More Board Review Help

Adam Brochert, MD, is a young physician who scored in the 99th percentile on Step 2 and has extensively researched the recent administrations of the USMLE. In addition to the Platinum Vignettes™, Dr. Brochert has written these best-selling USMLE reviews.

Crush the Boards

Crammed full of information from recent administrations of Step 2, this valuable review provides these features: high-yield information in a well-written, easily accessible format; complete coverage without being overwhelming; information is presented in the form it is asked about on Step 2; all subspecialty topics covered in Step 2 are addressed; text is filled with many helpful tables and illustrations; tips, insights, and guidance are offered on how best to prepare and what to expect.
2000 • 230 pages • illustrated • ISBN 1-56053-366-8 • $28 (US), $33 (outside US)

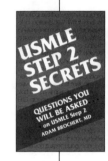

USMLE Step 2 Secrets

High-yield information taken from recent administrations of Step 2 is presented in the proven format of the best-selling Secrets Series®. Not just for memorization, Secrets presents a logical series of questions and answers that make you think about the answers and organize your thoughts. You will increase your confidence and guarantee your success on Step 2.
2000 • 265 pages • illustrated • ISBN 1-56053-451-6 • $35.95 (US), $40.95 (outside US)

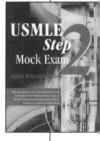

USMLE Step 2 Mock Exam

This valuable review is unique in the extent to which it simulates USMLE Step 2 conditions. Not only do the questions adhere to Step 2 clinical vignette formulations, but explanations ensure that you understand why your answer is right or wrong, a subject index allows you to focus on areas where you may need more study, and photos illustrate many of the conditions. Bottom line is that this popular review will help you master Step 2 material and increase your Step 2 scores. **USMLE STEP 2 MOCK EXAM also available in PDA format!**
2001 • 345 pages • illustrated • ISBN 1-56053-462-1 • $29 (US), $34 (outside US)

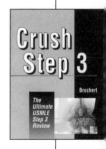

Crush Step 3

The author of the highly popular Crush the Boards presents this easy-to-use and effective high-yield review for Step 3. This review is perfect for the busy house officer who needs a review that hits all the important concepts and commonly tested topics in a concise format. The coverage also weaves in the kind of case-based scenarios that are one of the important keys to success in Step 3. It also contains the authors tips and guidance on how to prepare and what to expect. If you know the concepts in this book, you will Crush Step 3!
2001 • 225 pages • illustrated • ISBN 1-56053-484-2 • $29 (US), $34 (outside US)

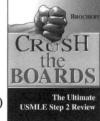

To order go to www.hanleyandbelfus.com